The Shoulder, Arm and Hand Syndrome

AUGUST L. SCHULTZ, D.C., Ph.C.

Printed by
Argus Printers
Stickney, S. Dak.

28/17/6

FOREWORD

In writing a book about as complicated an articulation as the shoulder joint, much consideration must be given to the many facets that present themselves. Symptoms in this extensive region are numerous, pathological conditions are many and nerve irritation caused by subluxations of the cervical and dorsal regions of the spine are no strangers to the chiropractic profession. These conditions cause the usual train of events: pain, reflex pain, neuritis, bursitis and many related painful symptoms. Subluxations of the ribs must also be remembered when dealing with the pain syndromes of the arm and shoulder regions. The dislocations and subluxations of the shoulder that may occur in numerous directions, presents in itself a vast amount of study concerning their correction and case management. The shoulder girdle consists of the clavicle, scapula and their articulations. Subluxations and dislocations of these articulations are often the offenders causing pain and reduced motility in the shoulder region. Certain muscles also enter into the picture and must be manipulated and specifically adjusted.

The writer does not intend to go extensively into the pathological area since this book is written from the standpoint of traumatic conditions. The doctor must decide, from his knowledge of diagnosis, the case history and x-rays, which of the techniques outlined will best be applicable to the case at hand. Along with the above outlined conditions, the writer will also show the techniques for the adjustment and case management of injuries to the elbow, wrist, thumb and fingers.

TABLE OF CONTENTS

Page

Chapter I
THE SHOULDER GIRDLE

The shoulder girdle is formed by the clavicle and scapula and, in front, it is completed by the upper end of the sternum which articulates with the medial end of the clavicle. Posteriorly the scapula is connected to the trunk by muscles. The clavicle is joined to the sternum by a double arthrodial joint. The two bones are separated by a cartilage, with one articulation behind the sternum and another between the cartilage and clavicle. The cartilage serves as an elastic buffer in case of shock received at the arm or shoulder. The joint permits the outer end of the clavicle to move up and down or forward and backward or any combination of these movements and also permitting slight rotation of the clavicle upon its axis. All movements of the shoulder girdle may be called movements of the scapula. The position of the clavicle does not permit independent movements. These movements always involve both bones, the clavicle moving in order to allow the scapula to assume its proper relation to the posterior chest wall.

The movements of the scapula may be classified as follows:

1. Backward toward the spinal column — adduction.
2. Sideways and forward away from the spinal column — abduction.
   This movement may extend through six inches or more being limited posteriorly by the contact of the two scapulae at the medial line and anteriorly by the resistance of the posterior muscles.
3. Upward movement of the entire scapula — elevation.
4. Downward movement — depression. The upward and downward movements may take place through a range of from four to five inches.
5. Rotation upward — rotation on a center to raise the acromion and turn the glenoid fossa upward.
6. Rotation downward. This is reverse rotation and may take place through an angle of 60 degrees or more. Rotation of the scapula is associated with all upward and downward movements of the arm. Since the clavicle is attached to

7

the sternum, which is comparatively stable, it is evident that the acromion must always move in a curve with the clavicle as the radius.

LIGAMENTS OF THE STERNOCLAVICULAR ARTICULATION

The ligaments of the sternoclavicular articulation are as follows:

1. The articular capsule
2. The anterior sternoclavicular
3. The posterior sternoclavicular
4. The interclavicular
5. The costoclavicular
6. The articular disc

THE ARTICULAR CAPSULE surrounds the articulation and varies in thickness and strength. In front and behind it is of considerable thickness, forming the anterior and posterior sternoclavicular ligaments. Above, and especially below, it is thin and partakes more of the characteristics of areolar than fibrous tissue.

THE ANTERIOR STERNOCLAVICULAR LIGAMENT is a broad band of fibers covering the anterior surface of the articulation. It is attached above to the upper and front part of the sternal end of the clavicle and below to the front and upper part of the manubrium sterni. This ligament is covered by the sternal portion of the sternocleidomastoideus.

THE POSTERIOR STERNOCLAVICULAR LIGAMENT is a similar band of fibers covering the posterior surface of the articulation. It is attached above to the upper and back part of the sternal end of the clavicle, passing obliquely downward and medialward. Then it is attached below to the manubrium sterni. It is in relation in front with the articular disc and the synovial membrane, and behind with the sternohyoideus and the sternothyroideus.

THE INTERCLAVICULAR LIGAMENT is a flattened band which varies considerably in form and size in different individuals. It passes in a curved direction from the upper part of the sternal end of one clavicle to that of the other. Also, it is attached to the upper margin of the sternum. It is in relation in front with the sternocleidomastoideus and behind with the sternothyroideus.

THE COSTOCLAVICULAR LIGAMENT is short, flat, strong and rhomboid in form. It is attached below to the upper and

8

medial part of the cartilage of the first rib and ascends obliquely backward and lateralward. It is attached above to the costal tuberosity on the undersurface of the clavicle and is in relation at the front with the tendon of origin of the subclavius, behind with the subclavian vein.

THE ARTICULAR DISC is a flat, nearly circular ligament and is interposed between the articular surfaces of the sternum and the clavicle. It is attached above to the upper and posterior borders of the articular surface of the clavicle, and below to the cartilage of the first rib near its junction with the sternum. There is further attachment by its circumference to the interclavicular and the anterior and posterior sternoclavicular ligaments. It is thicker at the circumference at its upper and back part, thinner at its center and it divides the joint into two cavities which are furnished with synovial membrane.

THE ACROMIOCLAVICULAR ARTICULATION

The acromioclavicular articulation is an arthrodial joint between the acromial end of the clavicle and the medial margin of the acromion of the scapula. Its ligaments are:

1. The articular capsule
2. The superior acromioclavicular
3. The inferior acromioclavicular
4. The articular disc
5. The coracoclavicular
6. The trapezoid
7. The conoid

THE ARTICULAR CAPSULE completely surrounds the articular margin. It is strengthened above and below by the superior and inferior acromioclavicular ligaments.

THE SUPERIOR ACROMIOCLAVICULAR LIGAMENT is quadrilateral, covering the superior part of the articulation, extending between the upper part of the acromio end of the clavicle and the adjoining part of the upper surface of the acromion. It is composed of parallel fibers which interlace with the aponeurosis of the trapezius and the deltoid below it. It is in contact with the articular disc when it is present.

THE INFERIOR ACROMIOCLAVICULAR LIGAMENT is somewhat thinner than the preceding one. It covers the underpart of the articulation and is attached to the adjoining surfaces of the two bones. It is in relationship above, in rare cases, with the articular disc and below, with the tendon of the supraspinatous.

THE ARTICULAR DISC is frequently absent in this articulation. When present, it generally partially separates the articular surfaces and occupies the upper part of the articulation.

THE CORACOCLAVICULAR LIGAMENT serves to connect the clavicle with the coracoid process of the scapula. It does not properly belong to this articulation but is usually described with it. It forms a most efficient means of retaining the clavicle in contact with the acromion. It consists of two fasciculae called the trapezoid and conoid ligaments.

THE TRAPEZOID LIGAMENT is composed of an anterior and a lateral fasciulus. It is broad, thin and quadrilateral, placed obliquely between the coracoid process and the clavicle. It is attached to the upper surface of the coracoid process and the clavicle and above to the oblique ridge of the under surface of the clavicle. Its anterior border is free while its posterior border is joined to the conoid ligament, the two forming by their junction an angle projecting backward.

THE CONOID LIGAMENT is composed of posterior and medial fasciculi. This is a dense band of fibers, conical in form, with its base directed upward. It is attached by its apex to the rough impression at the base of the coracoid process, medial to the trapezoid ligament; above, by its expanded base, to the coracoid tuberosity on the undersurface of the clavicle, and to a line proceeding medialward from it for 1.25 cm. These ligaments are in relation in front with the subclavius and deltoid; behind with the trapezius.

MOVEMENTS OF THE ACROMIOCLAVICULAR JOINT

The movements of this articulation are of two kinds, the one being a gliding motion of the articular end of the clavicle upon the acromion and the other being a rotation of the scapula forward and backward upon the clavicle. The extent of this rotation is limited by the two portions of the coroclavicular ligament, the trapezoid limiting the forward rotation and the conoid limiting the backward one.

The acromioclavicular joint has important functions in the movements of the upper extremity. It has been pointed out that

10

if there had been no joint between the clavicle and the scapula, and if there were no circular movement of the scapula upon the ribs (as in throwing the shoulder forward and backward), it would have been impossible to give a blow straight forward with the full force of the arm. With the combined force of the scapula, arm and forearm either bone can turn in a hinge-like manner upon a vertical axis. When the whole arch, formed by the clavicle and the scapula, rises and falls in elevation or depression of the shoulder, the joint between these bones enables the scapula to still maintain its lower part in contact with the ribs.

THE MUSCLES OF THE SHOULDER GIRDLE

The following seven muscles connect the shoulder girdle with the main skeleton, holding it in a normal position and giving rise to movements such as lifting, throwing, pushing, striking, etc. These movements involve both the arm and shoulder girdle. It is well to make a careful study of the individual actions of these muscles and they are as follows (Figs. 3 & 4):

1. The trapezius
2. The levator scapulae
3. The rhomboid major
4. The rhomboid minor
5. The serratus anterior
6. The pectoralis minor
7. The subclavius

THE TRAPEZIUS is a flat, triangular muscle covering the upper and back part of the neck and shoulder. *Origin:* the base of the skull, the ligamentum nuchae, the spinous processes of the vertebrae from the seventh cervical to the twelfth dorsal inclusive. *Insertion:* along a curved line following the outer third of the posterior border of the clavicle, the top of the acromion and the upper border of the spine of the scapula.

This important muscle is best studied in FOUR PARTS. PART ONE is a thin sheet of parallel fibers starting down from the base of the skull, then curving somewhat sideways and forward around the neck to the insertion of the clavicle. It is so thin and elastic that when it is relaxed, one or two fingertips can be pushed down between the outer third of the clavicle with ease, stretching the muscle before it and forming a small pocket; when it contracts, the fingers are lifted out and the pocket disappears. This enables

11

us to test the action of part one of the trapezius which is too thin to be seen and felt in the usual way.

PART TWO extends from the ligament of the neck to the acromion and is a much thicker and stronger sheet of fibers being tendinous at the origin and converging to the narrower insertion.

PART THREE is similar to part two, but stronger, and includes the fibers that arise from the seventh cervical and the upper three dorsal vertebrae. These converge somewhat into the insertion on the spine of the scapula.

PART FOUR, the lowest, is not as strong as the two middle portions but stronger than part one. The fibers converge from their origin on the lower dorsal vertebrae to join a short tendon attached to the small triangular space where the spine of the scapula ends near the vertebral border.

ACTION OF PART ONE OF THE TRAPEZIUS. It will lower the back of the skull and turn it to the side; since the skull is poised freely on a pivot at its base, this will tilt the chin up and turn the face to the opposite side. When part one of the right and left sides contract simultaneously, they will neutralize the tendency to rotate the head and will tilt the chin up with double force. With the head held still and the shoulder girdle free to move, contraction of this portion will evidently lift the clavicle and scapula, but with little force, because the muscle is thin and weak.

THE ACTION OF PART TWO. It will pull upward and inward, swinging the acromion on the sternal end of the clavicle as a center, and drawing it slightly backward or forward, depending upon the position of the neck and shoulder at the start of the movement.

THE ACTION OF PART THREE. Its pull is in a nearly horizontal line upon the spine of the scapula, drawing it in toward the spinal column; the posterior edge of the scapula will glide upon the posterior chest wall, while the swing of the clavicle will throw the acromion backward as the scapula is adducted.

ACTION OF PART FOUR: The pull of part four is such that it will draw the vertebral border of the scapula downward and slightly inward, the lower fibers pulling more directly downward.

When all the parts of the trapezius contract at once, it is important to notice that they act upon the upper, rather than the lower portion of the scapula, since they at the same time lift the acromion, adduct the spine and depress the vertebral border. They must, by their combined action, rotate the bone so as to turn the glenoid fossa upward rather than move the whole bone for any considerable distance in any direction. All parts of the trapezius come into action at the same time in raising the arms sideward, especially in raising the arm above shoulder level. No other bodily movements seem to employ the whole trapezius at once.

Nerve Supply: The trapezius is supplied by the accessory nerve and branches from the third and fourth cervical nerves.

THE LEVATOR SCAPULAE is situated at the back and side of the neck, beneath the first part of the trapezius. *Origin:* It arises by tendinous slips from the transverse processes of the atlas and axis and from the posterior tubercle and transverse processes of the third and fourth cervical vertebrae. *The Insertion* is the vertebral border of the scapula from its spine to the superior angle.

Action: If the head is fixed, the levator scapulae raise the medial angle of the scapulae. If the shoulder is fixed, the muscle inclines the neck to the corresponding side and rotates it in the same direction. The levator scapulae is an important support for the scapula in habitual posture, aiding the second part of the trapezius in holding it up to normal level. Subjects who have lost the use of the levator scapulae have the shoulder depressed.

Nerve Supply: This is from the third and fourth cervical nerves and frequently by a branch from the dorsal scapular.

THE RHOMBOID MAJOR — *Origin:* It arises by tendinous fibers from the spinous processes of the second, third, fourth and fifth cervical vertebrae and the supraspinal ligament. *Insertion:* It is inserted into a narrow, tendinous arch attached above to the lower part of the triangular surface at the root of the spine of the scapula and below to the inferior angle, the arch being connected to the vertebral border by a thin membrane.

THE RHOMBOID MINOR — *Origin:* It arises from the lower part of the ligamentum nuchae and from the spinous processes of the seventh cervical and first dorsal vertebrae. *Insertion:* It is inserted into the base of the triangular smooth surface at the root of the spine of the scapula. It is usually separated from the rhomboid major by a slight interval, however, the adjacent margins of the two muscles are occasionally united. *Actions:* The two muscles seem to have the same actions. The rhomboids carry the

13

inferior angle of the scapula backward and upward, thus producing a slight rotation of the scapula upon the side of the chest, the rhomboid major acting especially on the inferior angle of the scapula through the tendinous arch by which it is inserted. The rhomboidea acting together, with the middle and inferior fibers of the trapezius, will retract the scapula.

The rhomboids act powerfully in all downward movements of the arms, such as chopping with an axe, striking with a hammer, pulling on a rope and rowing a boat. Duchenne states that while the rhomboids are in contraction the subject cannot raise his arms above the shoulder level. Subjects who have lost the use of the rhomboids have the angle of the scapula projecting conspicuously from the back with a deep gutter beneath its edge, due to the pull of the muscles that attach to the upper part of the scapula. *The Nerve Supply* of the rhomboids is from the dorsal scapular nerve from the fifth cervical.

THE SERRATUS ANTERIOR is a thin, muscular sheath situated between the ribs and the scapula at the upper and lateral part of the chest. *Origin:* From the outer surface of the upper nine ribs at the side of the chest.

Structure: This muscle is in two separate parts, the upper and the lower. The upper part includes the fibers arising from the upper three ribs, diverging slightly to be inserted among the whole length of the scapula below its spine. The lower part is fan shaped, the fibers arising from the lower six attachments on the ribs, converging to be inserted together at the inferior angle of the scapula. The lower part is thicker and stronger than is the upper.

Action: The fibers of the serratus extend to nearly lengthwise of the ribs to exert much pull to move them unless the scapula is raised. Its upper fibers are well situated for drawing the scapula forward, as a whole, without rotation, as this motion takes place through the five or six inches of its extent. The swing of the clavicle upon the sternum will cause the acromion to move outward and then inward. The lower part of the muscle is in a position for vigorous rotation upward by drawing the inferior angle of the scapula forward. The lower fibers associate with the trapezius in turning the glenoid fossa upward. Subjects lacking the use of the serratus cannot lift the arm higher than the shoulder. When they try to do so, the vertebral border projects backward instead of lying close to the chest. *The Nerve Supply* of the serratus anterior is by the long thoracic which is derived from the fifth, sixth and seventh cervical nerves.

THE PECTORALIS MINOR: This is a small muscle located at the front of the upper chest and covered by the pectoralis major. *Origin:* From the outer surfaces of the third, fourth and fifth ribs at a point a little sideward from their junction with the costal cartilages. *The Insertion* is through groups of nearly parallel fibers that converge to join in a single tendon at the upper end of the coracoid process. *Action:* It may be said that the pectoralis minor acts in deep and forced breathing. It is placed in a position to help all movement involving abduction and downward rotation of the scapula which occurs in striking forward and downward as in chopping. *The Nerve Supply* of the pectoralis minor is from the eight cervical and first dorsal nerves through the medial anterior and thoracic nerves.

THE SUBCLAVIUS: This is a small muscle located beneath the clavicle. *Origin:* From the upper surface of the first rib where it joins its cartilage. *Insertion:* It inserts into a groove extending along the middle half of the underside of the clavicle. *Action:* The subclavius depresses the shoulder by carrying it downward and forward. *Nerve Supply:* The subclavius is supplied by a filament from the fifth and sixth cervical nerves.

SUMMARY OF THE MECHANICS OF THE SHOULDER GIRDLE

The shoulder girdle is so freely movable that its habitual position depends upon its relative tension of the seven muscles just described, together with some influence produced by two others that act indirectly on it through the arm, namely the triceps and biceps.

THE STERNOCLAVICULAR JOINT

The medial end of the clavicle is rounded and bulbous and articulates with the sternum in a shallow socket. About half of the medial end of the clavicle rides above the slanting sternal notch. Some instability and a tendency to dislocation to the medial aspect results from this arrangement. It is guarded against injury by an articular disc, or check ligament, attached in a roundabout way from the top across the end to a point underneath the clavicle. Force applied to the lateral portion of the shoulder is transmitted along the clavicle and is snubbed or checked by the action and attachment of this ligament. The margins blend, front and back,

15

with the capsular expansions, strengthening the attachment of the central cartilaginous disc. The intra-articular disc may be torn or damaged, leading to internal derangement of this joint similar in manner to the meniscus injuries encountered in the knee. The anterior aspect of the joint is covered by fibers of the sternomastoid muscle. Behind there is a thick pad of muscle fibers from the sternohyoid and sternothyroid which cushions and protects the great vessels (Fig. 1).

THE CORACOCLAVICULAR MECHANISM (CONOID AND TRAPEZOID LIGAMENTS)

This is described on page 27.

THE ACROMIOCLAVICULAR JOINT

The acromioclavicular joint is the third joint mechanism associated with the clavicle. Normally, it is quite stable, being supported by the capsular ligament. The clavicle is supported by a downward pull through the coracoclavicular ligament. The joint surface is normally vertical but obliquity is often found without causing symptoms. Past middle life, roughening of the clavicle, spur formation or narrowing of the joint may be found. Depending somewhat on the case history of injury and the occupation of the subject, x-ray examination will reveal this condition.

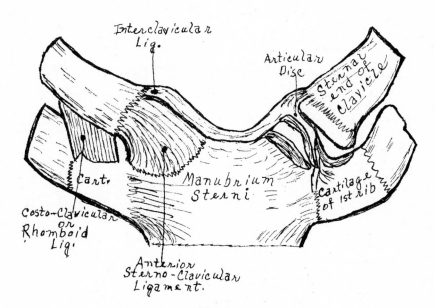

Fig. 1
STERNOCLAVICULAR ARTICULATION
Anterior View   (Gray)

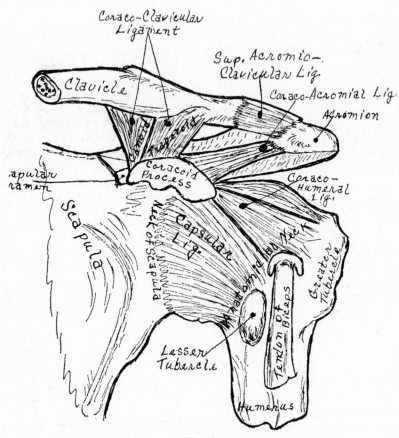

Fig. 2
**LEFT SHOULDER AND ACROMIOCLAVICULAR JOINTS
AND PROPER SCAPULAR LIGAMENTS** (Gray)

Chapter II
THE SHOULDER JOINT

THE HUMERAL ARTICULATION

The shoulder joint is a ball and socket articulation and the bones entering into its formation are the head of the humerus and the shallow glenoid cavity of the scapula, an arrangement that allows considerable movement. The articulation is protected against displacement by the tendons which surround it. The ligaments do not maintain the joint in its position, since, when they alone remain, the humerus can be separated to a considerable extent from the glenoid cavity. Their use is to limit the amount of movement. The joint is protected from above by an arch formed by the coracoid process, the acromion, and the coracoacromial ligament. The articular cartilage on the head of the humerus is thicker at the center than at the circumference, the reverse being the case with the articular cartilage of the glenoid cavity.

The ligaments of the shoulder are as follows:
1. The articular capsule
2. The coracohumeral
3. The glenohumeral
4. The transverse humeral
5. The glenoid labrum

THE ARTICULAR CAPSULE completely encircles the articulation, being attached above to the circumference of the glenoid cavity, below to the anatomical neck of the humerus. It is thicker above and below than elsewhere and is so remarkably loose and lax that it has no action in keeping the bones in contact. It allows the two bones to separate from each other by more than 2.5 cm. It is strengthened above by the supraspinatous, below by the long head of the biceps brachii, behind by the tendons of the infrapinatous and teres minor, and in front by the tendons of the subscapularis.

There are usually three openings in the capsule, one anteriorly below the coracoid process which establishes a communication between the joint and the bursa beneath the tendon of the subscapularis. The second opening is not constant, and when present, is at the posterior part where the opening sometimes exists between the joint and bursal sac, under the tendon of the infraspinatous. The third one is between the tubercles of the humerus, allowing for the passage of the long tendon of the biceps brachii.

THE CORACOHUMERAL LIGAMENT is a broad band which strengthens the upper part of the capsule. It arises from the lateral border of the coracoid process and passes obliquely downward and lateralward to the front of the greater tubercle of the humerus and blending with the tendon of the supraspinatous. This ligament is intimately united to the capsule by its posterior and lower borders. The anterior and upper borders present a free edge which overlaps the capsule (Fig. 2).

THE GLENOHUMERAL LIGAMENTS. In addition to the coracohumeral ligament, three supplemental bands, which are named the glenohumeral ligaments, strengthen the capsule. One on the medial side of the joint passes from the medial edge of the glenoid cavity to the lower part of the lesser tubercle of the humerus. A second band at the lower part of the joint extends from the under edge of the glenoid cavity to the under part of the anatomical neck of the humerus. A third band at the upper part of the joint is fixed above to the apex of the glenoid cavity close to the root of the coracoid process, passes downward along the medial edge of the tendon to the biceps brachii, and then is attached below to a small depression above the lesser tubercle of the humerus. The capsule is also strengthened in front by two bands derived from the tendons of the pectoralis major and teres major respectively.

THE TRANSVERSE HUMERAL LIGAMENT is a broad band passing from the lesser to the greater tubercle of the humerus. It is also united to that portion of bone which lies above the epiphyseal line. It converts the intertubercular groove into a canal.

THE GLENOID LABRUM or glenoid ligament is a fibrocartilaginous rim attached around the margin of the glenoid cavity. It is a triangular section, the base being fixed to the circumference of the cavity, while the free edge is thin and sharp. It is continuous with the tendon of the long head of the biceps brachii, which in turn, gives off two fasciculi to blend with the fibrous tissue of the labrum. It deepens the articular cavity and protects the edge of the bone.

THE SYNOVIAL MEMBRANE

The synovial membrane is reflected from the margin of the glenoid cavity over the labrum. It is then reflected over the inner surface of the capsule and covers the lower part and sides of the anatomical neck of the humerus, as far as the articular cartilage on the head of the bone. The tendon of the long head of the biceps brachii passes through the capsule and is enclosed in a tubular sheath of the synovial membrane which is reflected upon it from the summit of the glenoid cavity and is continued around the tendon into the intertubercular groove as far as the surgical neck of the humerus.

The shoulder joint is capable of every variety of movement; flexion, extension, abduction, adduction, circumduction and rotation. The most striking peculiarities of this joint are:

1. The large size of the head of the humerus when compared with the depth of the glenoid cavity.

2. The looseness of the capsule of the articulation.

3. The intimate connection of the capsule with the tendons of the muscles attached to the head of the humerus.

4. The peculiar relationship of the tendons of the long head of the biceps brachii to the joint. It also acts as one of the ligaments of this articulation. It helps retain the head close to the glenoid cavity, thus guarding against upward displacement.

THE BURSAE AND THEIR RELATIONSHIP TO THE SHOULDER JOINT

1. A constant bursa is situated between the tendon of the subscapularis muscle and the capsule. It communicates with the synovial cavity through an opening in front of the capsule.

2. A bursa which occasionally communicates with the joint is sometimes found between the tendons of the infraspinatous and the capsule.

3. A large bursa exists between the under surface of the deltoid and the capsule but does not communicate with the joint. This bursa is prolonged under the acromion and the coracoacromial ligament and intervenes between these structures and the capsule.

4. A large bursa is situated on the summit of the acromion.

5. A bursa is frequently found between the coracoid process and the capsule.

6. A bursa exists beneath the coracobrachialis.

7. A bursa lies between the teres major and the long head of the triceps brachii.

8. One is placed in front of, and another behind the tendon of the latissimus dorsi.

MUSCLES ACTING UPON THE SHOULDER JOINT

Movements of the shoulder articulation are produced by nine muscles, along with some assistance from the triceps, which acts upon the shoulder joint with one of its parts while its main action is upon the elbow.

The nine are conveniently placed in three groups of three muscles each. Three of the nine are large muscles and are placed above, in front and at the rear. With each of these goes a small associate muscle and a rotator of the humerus.

	Muscle	*Small Associates*	*Rotators*
ABOVE	Deltoid	Supraspinatous	Infraspinatous
FRONT	Pectoralis Major	Coracobrachialis	Subscapularis
REAR	Latissimus	Teres Major	Teres Minor

THE DELTOID

The deltoid is a large, thick, triangular muscle which covers the shoulder joint in front, behind and laterally. *Origin:* It arises from the anterior border and upper surfaces of the lateral third of the clavicle, from the lateral margin and upper surface of the acromion and from the lower lip of the posterior border of the spine of the scapula. *Insertion:* It inserts in an area on the outer surface of the humerus, somewhat above the middle portion of the bone.

Structure: There are three parts, namely front, middle and posterior. The front and posterior portions are simple penniforms while the middle is more complex. The tendon of insertion divides into five strands near the humerus; the outer two placed in the front and rear, receive fibers of the front and rear portions of the muscle which arises directly from the bones above; the middle has four tendons of origin, passing from the acromion, and the three tendons of insertion passing up from below alternate between them; the muscular fibers of the middle portion pass diagonally across between the seven tendons. The result of the arrangement is that the middle part has more power and a lesser extent of contraction that the other two parts.

Action: The deltoid raises the arm from the side to bring it at right angles with the trunk. Its anterior fibers, assisted by the pectoralis, draws the arm forward. The posterior fibers, aided by the teres major and the latissimus dorsi, draw the arm backward.

Nerve Supply: The deltoid is supplied by the fifth and sixth cervical nerves through the axillary nerve.

Loss of one or more of the three portions of the deltoid interferes seriously with all movement involving the elevation of the arm. Subjects with this defect have difficulty in feeding and dressing themselves. Loss of the use of the posterior deltoid makes it impossible to place the arm behind the body at the waistline. If loss of use is sustained to the front part of the deltoid, the subject cannot bring his hand up to his face or put his hat on without bending the head forward. If the front or middle portion is affected, the arm cannot be lifted above the shoulder level in any direction. Few muscles are so important to the common movements of the arm as is the deltoid.

THE SUPRASPINATOUS

The supraspinatous is a thick, triangular muscle filling the supraspinatous fossa and is covered in part by the trapezius. *Origin:* It originates from the inner two thirds of the supraspinatous fossa. *Insertion:* It inserts into the top of the greater tuberosity of the humerus.

Action: The supraspinatous pulls on the humerus with a short power arm at a great angle. It joins the humerus above the axis and is powerful enough to lift the arm to its own full height, even when the deltoid power is lost, though it soon fatigues when so much stress is placed upon it. It pulls the head of the humerus directly into the socket thus preventing upward displacement. For this reason, a person who has lost the use of the supraspinatous cannot do much work involving elevation of the arms. *Nerve Supply:* The nerve supply is from the fifth and sixth cervical nerves through the suprascapular nerve.

THE PECTORALIS MAJOR

This is a large, fan shaped muscle lying immediately beneath the skin over the chest. *Origin:* It originates from the inner two-thirds of the anterior border of the clavicle, the whole length of the sternum and the cartilages of the first six ribs near the junction of the sternum. *Insertion:* It is inserted by a flat tendon, about three inches wide, into a ridge that forms the outer border of the bicipital groove of the humerus, extending from just below the tuberosity, nearly down to the insertion of the deltoid muscle.

Action: If the arm has been raised by the deltoid, the pectoralis major will, cojointly with the latissimus dorsi and teres major, depress it to the sides of the chest. If acting alone, it adducts and draws the arm forward, bringing it across the front of the chest and at the same time, rotates the arm inward.

THE CORACOBRACHIALIS

This is a small muscle named from its attachments and is located deep beneath the deltoid and pectoralis major on the front and inner side of the arm. *Insertion:* It is inserted into the inner surface of the humerus.

Action: The coracobrachialis draws the humerus forward and medialward. It also assists in retaining the head of the humerus in contact with the glenoid cavity. *Nerve Supply:* The nerve supply is received from the seventh cervical nerve and the musculocutaneous nerve which perforates the muscle.

THE LATISSIMUS DORSI

The latissimus dorsi is a broad, triangular muscle which covers the lumbar area and the lower half of the thoracic region. It is gradually contracted into a narrow, flat tendon at its insertion into the humerus. *Origin:* It originates from the spinous processes of the lower six dorsal vertebrae and all of the lumbars, the crest of the ilium and the lower three ribs. *Insertion:* It inserts into the bottom of the bicipital groove of the humerus by a flat tendon attached parallel to the upper three quarters of the insertion of the pectoralis major.

Action: The movements effected by this great muscle are numerous, as may be conceived by its attachments. The latissimus dorsi is situated so that it will pull the arm downward toward the side from any position of elevation. The lower fibers are in a position to act to the best advantage when the arm is high, pulling at a right angle when it is near the horizontal plane, and in so doing, they tend to depress the acromion. Their short lever arm makes the fibers adapted to speed rather than power. When the arm has been lowered to forty-five degrees, the upper fibers

24

pull at a better leverage than the lower fibers. This tends to adduct the arm and also the scapula. The muscle, when working as a whole, has its best leverage at about forty-five degrees of arm elevation. When it pulls at a right angle, it pulls the arm to the rear of the lateral plane. Its insertion on the front of the humerus makes it an inward rotor and its position at the rear of the trunk enables it to turn farther than the pectoralis major. Isolated action of the latissimus produces what we would expect, namely the upper fibers adduct the scapula so accurately and strongly that this places it among the muscles that maintain normal posture of the shoulder girdle. The lower fibers contract with the arm at the side and draw the head of the humerus down from the socket as far as the capsule and associated tendons will permit.

Nerve Supply: The latissimus dorsi is supplied by the sixth, seventh and eighth cervical nerves through the thoraco-dorsal nerve.

THE TERES MAJOR

The teres major is a thick, somewhat flattened muscle lying along the axillary border of the scapula. *Origin:* It originates from the external surface of the lower end of the axillary border. *Insertion:* It inserts into the ridge that forms the inner border of the bicipital groove of the humerus, parallel to the middle half of the insertion of the pectoralis major.

Action: This muscle is in a position to pull the humerus and axillary border together, and therefore it is the most direct antagonist of the deltoid. It pulls at a right angle when the humerus has been moved from the side to about forty-five degrees. The position of its insertion enables it to rotate the arm inward. *Nerve Supply:* This muscle is supplied by the fifth and sixth cervical nerves through the subscapular nerve.

THE SUBSCAPULARIS

Origin: It originates from the whole inner surface of the scapula, next to the ribs. *Insertion:* The subscapularis inserts into the lesser tuberosity of the humerus. *Action:* This muscle rotates the head of the humerus inward. When the arm is raised, it draws the humerus forward and downward. It is a powerful defense to the front of the shoulder joint, preventing displacement to the head of the humerus. *Nerve Supply:* The subscapularis is supplied by the fifth and sixth cervical nerves through the upper and lower subscapularis nerves.

Summary of the Mechanics of the Glenohumeral Joint

What is commonly considered the shoulder joint is in reality three distinct articulating mechanisms, namely the acromio-humeral, the glenohumeral and the bicipital arrangement. All three mechanisms are intimately related so that injury or disease of one interferes with the action of the others, or they may all be directly involved.

The central mechanism of the shoulder is the ball and socket arrangement. The others are auxiliary and aid in producing the wide range of mobility of this articulation, allowing it to function in many planes. The socket is a shallow, pear shaped fulcrum on which a sphenoid rides. The medial rim is indented by the subscapularis tendon as it passes to the humerus. The head of the humerus bears the brunt of any joint damage and is the moving part that has the largest cartilage covered area.

THE SUBACROMIAL BURSA

On the top of the humerus and under the acromion lies an important and extensive bursa, namely the subacromial, the sole purpose of which is to enhance the range of shoulder movement. It functions as a second joint for the humeral head by providing the lubricating mechanism which in turn allows movements to the front, above shoulder level and also makes it possible for the humeral head to roll under the arch and yet rotate on its long axis.

The bursa is hung from the underside of the acromion, the coracoacromio ligament and the undersurface of the deltoid muscle. It extends under the coracoid, over the subscapularis and the muscles that attach to the coracoid process. Its base covers most of the greater tuberosity and extends medially over the rotor cuff. Normally the bursa is thin walled and does not communicate with the shoulder joint. The rotor cuff is the floor, and the bursa usually extends somewhat behind the muscle-tendon junction. Its position and function make it vulnerable to wear and tear damage since it cushions the tuberosity from impinging on the arch. The floor may be torn in a cuff rupture which will result in folds and a thickening of the walls. This is the bursa that is involved in cases of shoulder bursitis and it is sometimes also called the subdeltoid bursa (Fig. 3 & 18).

As has been shown previously, the shoulder is endowed with many bursae. Their purpose is to lubricate the points of stress and friction, and the most important of these are the subacromial and the synovial sleeve on the biceps. Bursitis will be discussed at a later point.

THE MECHANICS OF THE BICIPITAL TENDON

Through both the acromiohumeral and glenohumeral joint, there passes an accessory ligament. This is the long head of the biceps and it enters the joint anteriorly in the synovial sleeve, passing under a short transverse intertubercular ligament, then passing across the head. It helps to retain the head close to the glenoid cavity thus helping to guard against upward displacement. With the arm extended, the head of the humerus slips out from the overhanging coracoacromial arch. It is in this position that the biceps tendon is the principal structure in preventing dislocation. The tendon is retained in position by the transverse humeral ligament and the adjacent fibers of the rotor cuff. In external rotation and abduction, this supporting mechanism is put under strain and the lesser tuberosity becomes a fulcrum as the head passes underneath the tendon. In accidents where injury of the shoulder takes place in these positions, the transverse ligament and adjacent capsule may rupture, allowing the biceps tendon to slip out medially (Fig. 2 & 26).

THE CORACOCLAVICULAR MECHANISM

This is the suspensory ligament of the upper extremity and serves as a joint, producing a fulcrum near the lateral end of the clavicle for swinging the shoulder girdle. The ligament suspends the scapula by the protruding coracoid process to the under surface of the clavicle. The scapula and arm swing on this arrangement. Anatomically this is made up of two parts, namely the trapezoid and conoid ligaments, but functionally they act as a single ligament. The direction of these fibers is such that they resist downward and inward slipping of the scapula, and with the clavicle holding the arm outward, these ligaments may be torn. In an acromioclavicular dislocation, the neurovascular bundle running just below it, may be damaged. Fig. 2.

THE MECHANICS OF THE ACROMIOCLAVICULAR JOINT

The role of the acromioclavicular joint is far far more important than the credit given it in the past. The movements which occur are flexion, extension and circumduction. Bateman states

27

as follows: "The contribution to circumduction is important. Movement occurs during the early part of the second 90 degrees, with the acromion dipping or sliding on the clavicle, and does not start until the arm reaches the right angle. Appreciation of the timing of this action is important in recognizing acromioclavicular disturbance as apart from glenohumeral disorder. The pain in acromioclavicular arthritis occurs after 90 degrees is reached, in contrast to the pain in degenerative tendinitis which develops before this point."

The Ligaments of the Scapula

The ligaments of the scapula are as follows (Fig. 2):
1. The coracoacromial
2. The superior transverse
3. The inferior transverse

THE CORACOACROMIAL LIGAMENT is a strong triangular band extending between the coracoid process and the acromion. It is attached by its apex to the summit of the acromion just in front of the articular surface of the clavicle; and by its broad base to the whole length of the lateral border of the coracoid process. This ligament, together with the coracoid process of the acromion, forms a vault for the protection of the head of the humerus. It is in relation above, with the clavicle and the under surface of the deltoid; below, with the tendon of the supraspinatous where a bursa has been interposed. Its lateral border is continuous with a dense lamina that passes beneath the deltoid and upon the tendons of the supraspinatous and the infraspinatous.

THE SUPERIOR TRANSVERSE LIGAMENT converts the scapular notch into a foramen. It is a thin and flat fasciculus, narrower at the middle than at the extremities, attached by one end to the base of the coracoid process, by the other end to the medial end of the scapular notch. The suprascapular nerve runs through this foramen. The transverse scapular vessels cross over the ligament. The ligament is sometimes ossified.

THE INFERIOR TRANSVERSE LIGAMENT is a weak, membranous band situated behind the neck of the scapula and stretching from the lateral border of the spine of the scapula to the margin of the glenoid cavity. It forms an arch under which the transverse scapular vessels and suprascapular nerve enters the infraspinatous fossa.

THE MECHANICS OF THE SCAPULO-THORACIC AREA

The contribution of the scapula to shoulder function is one of the most remarkable in body mechanics. It acts as a base or platform for the upper extremity, yet takes part in the movements of the shoulder girdle, and in addition, it aids the movement of the glenohumeral joint. The movements that are possible at the scapulo-thoracic joint are abduction, elevation, depression and rotation. All of these movements are accomplished by the flat scapular movements on the posterior chest wall. Since the same

29

pathway is constantly used, it is simple to see that irregularities are apt to occur from constant wear and tear. This very important area directly and indirectly affects many shoulder conditions and will be discussed in the adjustive techniques.

ABDUCTION OR LATERAL MOVEMENTS OF THE SCAPULA: The scapula moves around the posterior chest wall and in many individuals it is to a distance of four to five inches. The maximum is reached when the arm is flexed across the chest. The muscles involved in this action are the pectoralis minor and the serratus anterior along with the pectoralis major, though this last mentioned is to a lesser degree. The movement follows a curved course on the chest wall from behind the posterior angle of the rib to the front. A weak serratus will interfere with this action.

ADDUCTION OR MEDIAL MOVEMENT OF THE SCAPULA: From the relaxed position, one scapula may be moved toward the other, stopping just lateral to the posterior spinous processes. As this occurs, the muscles between the two scapulae tend to bulge, thus resisting the action. Adduction is accomplished by the trapezius, the rhomboid major and the rhomboid minor pulling on the medial border of the spine of the scapula. Note the important muscles attached to it as shown in Fig. 74.

ELEVATION OF THE SCAPULA: The scapula is elevated on the posterior chest wall in a movement such as shrugging the shoulders. It moves upward approximately two and one-half inches, shifting slightly lateralward in its upward movement. This movement is accomplished by the levator scapulae and the upper portions of the trapezius. Movement also occurs at the sternoclavicular joint.

DEPRESSION OF THE SCAPULA: The point of the shoulder may be lowered to a small degree and it shifts downward only about one-half of an inch. However, most of this movement is accomplished by a downward rotation rather than depression. This movement is accomplished by the action of the lower fibers of the serratus anterior with some help from the pectoralis minor and the subclavian.

ROTATION OF THE SCAPULO-THORACIC JOINT: In addition to the movement in the vertical and horizontal directions, the scapular rotation is wheel-like. Attached to the posterior chest wall, the center of the wheel is just below the middle of the spine. This motion is associated with the raising and lower-

30

ing of the arm. During the first thirty degrees of circumduction, the scapula is fixed. However, at this point it starts to tilt upward so the base of the glenoid follows the head of the humerus, and from here to the completion of the arc of elevation, the scapula rotates sixty degrees. This movement is accomplished by the serratus anterior and the trapezius. The pull of the levator scapulae, both rhomboids and the pectoralis minor return it to its normal position. Figs. 3 & 4.

ACTIONS OF THE IMPORTANT SHOULDER MUSCLES

It may seem to the doctor reading this book that the writer has gone into a great deal of repetition in the study of the muscles and their actions in the shoulder and its adjacent structures. This is done for several reasons. First, these muscles are of paramount importance in the diagnosis and correction of the many shoulder irregularities.

Second, in order to become adept in the recognition and correction of the cases that appear in your offices, it is necessary to have a foundation, not only in anatomy, but also in kinesiology and the research of such recognized authorities as Bateman, Judovitch, Bates and others. Since it is, for the most part, impossible for the busy doctor to take the time to ferret out the salient information that is necessary for the correction of these cases, it is the writer's hope that he has accomplished this tedious task for him.

As we get into the techniques of muscle manipulation and shoulder and muscle adjusting, it is necessary to know the attachments, origins, insertions, actions and nerve supply of these muscles. The shoulder girdle is an architectural marvel with its intricate and powerful muscular systems which are called upon to suspend and stabilize the structure as well as to provide the power of movement. In the lower extremity, one of the most important functions is that of upright stability and this is enhanced by the bony structures of the parts. In the shoulder this is not true and stability has been sacrificed to increase mobility and therefore the burden upon the muscular system has been considerably increased.

THE ACTION OF THE TRAPEZIUS AND SERRATUS ANTERIOR: As has been stated previously, the trapezius is really a muscular system of four parts that produce different movements. The muscle as a whole braces the shoulder backwards, and the

31

upper fibers help to suspend the shoulder girdle in the static role. They also shrug the shoulder and contribute to the balance and support of the head and shoulder, exerting a continuous tension and backward pull on the head and shoulders. The upper central fibers, by their attachment to the acromion, pull the whole shoulder girdle upward and inward.

The lower portion of the trapezius plays an important action in circumduction of the arm. This portion of the muscle, along with the serratus anterior fixes the scapula to the chest wall so that it cannot slip sideways or rotate and in this way a base is provided for the contraction of the deltoid. The serratus anterior assists in stabilizing the base of the upper extremity of the chest and acts as a powerful rotator. In the movement of circumduction, any weakness in the serratus anterior leaves an insecurely fixed scapula, thereby weakening the action of the deltoid.

ACTION OF THE DELTOID: The deltoid is a multi-pennate muscle with the fibers arranged so that a diagonal pull is produced. This structure allows a large number of fibers to contract, producing a great amount of strength. The anterior and posterior parts are composed of parallel fibers to enable free range in acts of flexion and extension. The most important action of this muscle is in the movements of abduction and circumduction. After the scapula becomes stationary and the head of the humerus fixed or stabilized, the deltoid swings the arm outward and upward. In this action the deltoid contracts as soon as the scapula is fixed and continues to lift the arm outward and upward on its base. The middle portion of the muscle initiates the movement and later, as the arm ascends above the head, the anterior and posterior parts join in also.

In swinging the arm, the deltoid acts to control the movement of the upper arm during the backward swing, and it also controls forward swinging during the movement. The anterior deltoid pulls the humerus forward with the aid of the pectoralis major for the delivery of a powerful punch. The muscle system of the deltoid is enhanced at its periphery by the pectoralis on one side and the teres major and minor on the other. In strong forward flexion, such as in pitching, the anterior deltoid is supported by the pectoralis major while the teres major and minor muscles support the posterior deltoid.

The Rotor Cuff

THE ROTOR CUFF MUSCLES are a very important group and enter into the picture in many shoulder injuries. This group includes the supraspinatous, the infraspinatous, the teres minor and the subscapularis which all contribute to certain vital movements. The group should be considered as a unit rather than separate, individual muscles because their insertions blend into a common tendon through which all of the action is directed.

THE SUPERIOR PORTION OF THE CUFF: The supraspinatous controls this part of the cuff by applying tension through a short lever to the top of the humerus. As the muscle contracts, it depresses the humeral head so that it moves downward and is stabilized in the glenoid cavity. This situation, along with the application of force through a longer lever by the powerful deltoid, and the stabilization by the cuff, produces a steady fulcrum allowing the deltoid to act efficiently.

THE POSTERIOR PORTION OF THE CUFF: This segment of the cuff is largely controlled by the infraspinatous with contributions from the teres minor. The infraspinatous is a bulky muscle with a much larger cross-section than the supraspinatous and it exerts a strong pull. The fleshy fibers extend well up into the capsule and the line of pull is downward. It can also act as an extensor in the horizontal plane or externally rotate the humerus.

The combination of depression, extension and external rotation is an important contribution to swinging the greater tuberosity underneath the coracoacromial arch during abduction. When there is interference with this mechanism, such as in rupture or degeneration, circumduction is obstructed as the humerus jams the overhanging arch. The external rotation of the muscle is also aided by the fixation of the scapula by the rhomboids. With the scapula flattened against the back, the humerus can be more effectively rotated.

THE ANTERIOR PORTION OF THE CUFF: The subscapularis controls this portion of the cuff and is a broad, flat muscle covering the anterior surface of the scapula. The tendon is adherent to the capsule in front and below. The subscapularis acts as an internal rotator and adductor while at the same time exerting a downward pull which depresses the head of the humerus. Thus it aids the stabilizing action of the supraspinatous and the infraspinatous. It also acts as a ligament in helping to maintain the head of the humerus in the glenoid cavity.

All of the rotator muscles act through a common tendon which is constantly under tension on the superior, posterior and anterior aspects of the shoulder and this may initiate wear and tear damage. The superior portion of the cuff is in constant tension by dutifully maintaining the humeral head in proper relation with the glenoid cavity (Fig. 20).

STATIC FUNCTION OF THE SHOULDER GIRDLE: The bones act as levers for the transmission of force and the ligaments supplement this action and contribute suspension and stability in addition to the part played by the joints and the muscular system. In a fall on the outstretched hand, force is transmitted from the hand and forearm to the humerus, then to the scapula and clavicle. The scapula receives the force through the glenoid cavity and is transferred to the clavicle through the coracoclavicular ligament. Since the impact usually occurs with the arm abducted, the overhanging acromion is rarely fractured, however, the clavicle often is and the shoulder shares in the impact. With the arm pulling into adduction, the acromion and clavicle transmit the major force so that either acromioclavicular dislocations or clavicular fracture may occur.

THE MUSCLES OF THE ARM

The four muscles of the arm are as follows:

1. The coracobrachialis
2. The biceps brachii
3. The brachialis
4. The triceps brachii

THE CORACOBRACHIALIS has been described with the humeral rotators on page 35 (Fig. 3).

THE BICEPS BRACHII is a prominent muscle on the front side of the upper arm having two separate places of origin. ORIGIN 1: The outer, or long head, arises from the scapula at the top of the glenoid bursa and the tendon passes over the head of the humerus and blends with the capsular ligament of the shoulder joint. ORIGIN 2: The inner, or short head, arises from the coracoid process. *Insertion:* Both parts insert into the bicipital tuberosity of the radius. *Structure:* The tendon of the long

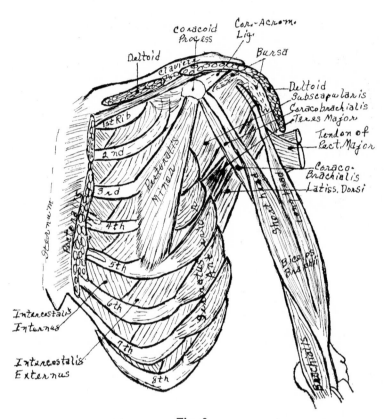

Fig. 3

**DEEP MUSCLES OF THE CHEST AND FRONT OF ARM
WITH AUXILIARIES** (Gray)

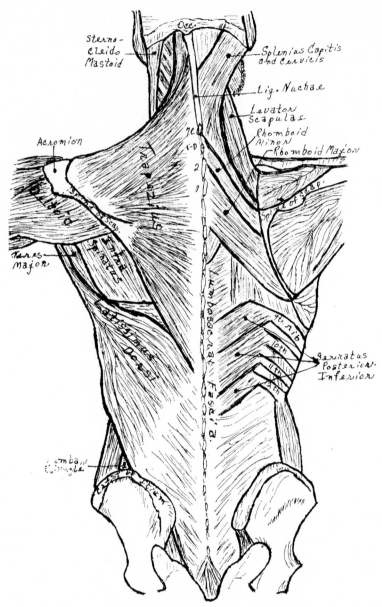

Fig. 4
**MUSCLES CONNECTING THE UPPER EXTREMITY TO
THE VERTEBRAL COLUMN**   (Gray)

36

head is long and slender and lies in the bicipital groove of the humerus, becoming muscular at the lower end of the groove. The tendon of the inner head is shorter, the mucular fibers of the two parts being of equal length. The tendon of insertion is flattened as it joins the muscle and passes up as a septum between the two parts and receives the fibers in a penniform manner from both sides.

Action: The biceps is in a position to act on three articulations, namely the shoulder, elbow and forearm. Tension on the long head aids in holding the head of the humerus in its socket and the short head acts with it to lift the humerus lengthwise. Both parts act to flex the elbow. When the hand is placed in extreme pronation, the bicipital tuberosity of the radius is turned inward and downward, wrapping the tendon of the biceps more than half way around the bone. Contraction of the muscle will tend to unwrap it and thus supinate the hand. Both the flexing and supinating actions of the biceps will take place to the best mechanical advantage when the arm is half flexed. *Nerve Supply:* The biceps brachii is supplied by the musculo-cutaneous nerve and from the fifth and sixth cervical nerves (Fig. 11).

THE BRACHIALIS covers the front of the elbow joint and the lower half of the humerus. *Origin:* It arises from the lower half of the front of the humerus commencing above at the insertion of the deltoid which it embraces by two angular processes. Its fibers converge into a thick tendon. *Insertion:* It inserts into the tuberosity of the ulna and the rough depression on the anterior surface of the coronoid process.

THE TRICEPS is on the posterior side of the upper arm and, as its name implies, it has three separate points of origin. *Origin 1:* The long head arises by a flattened tendon from the infraglenoid tuberosity of the scapula being blended at its upper part with the capsule of the shoulder joint. The muscular fibers pass downward between the other heads of the muscle and join them in the tendon of insertion. *Origin 2:* The lateral head arises from the posterior surface of the body of the humerus between the insertion of the teres minor and the upper part of the groove for the radial nerve, and from the lateral border of the humerus and the lateral intermuscular septum. The fibers from this origin converge toward the tendon of insertion. *Origin 3:* The medial head arises from the posterior surface of the body of the humerus below the groove for the radial nerve. It is narrow and pointed above, and extends from the insertion of the teres major to within 2.5 cm of the trochlea. It also arises from the medial border of the humerus and from the back of the whole length of the medial intermuscular septum. Some of the fibers are directed downward to the olecranon and others converge to the tendon of insertion. *Action:* The triceps is the great extensor muscle of the forearm. It is the direct antagonist of the biceps brachii and the brachialis. When the arm is extended, the long head of the muscle may assist the teres major and the latissimus dorsi in drawing the humerus backward and in adducting it to the thorax. The long head supports the underpart of the shoulder joint. *Nerve Supply:* The triceps brachii is supplied by the seventh and eighth cervical nerves through the radial nerve (Fig. 11).

Chapter III

THE ELBOW

THE ELBOW JOINT

The arm has a hinge joint at the elbow and a rotary union of the radius and ulna at the forearm.

The elbow is a typical hinge joint, the humerus articulating closely with the ulna and but slightly with the radius. The movements are flexion and extension, these taking place through an angle, varying in different subjects from one hundred and twenty to one hundred and fifty degrees. Extension is limited by contact of the olecranon process of the ulna against the side of the humerus. Flexion is limited by contact of the muscles on the front of the arm. Some individuals can over-extend the arm at the elbow while others cannot fully extend it, this difference being due mainly to occupation, habitual position of the joint and variations in the laxness of the ligaments. The capsule of the joint is reinforced by strong bands of connective tissue on the outer and inner sides.

THE RADIO-ULNAR UNION is a double pivot joint with the radius rotating in a ligamentous ring at the elbow and the lower ends of the two bones describing a semicircle around each other at the wrist. The ulna cannot rotate at the elbow and the radius cannot rotate at the wrist, yet by means of the peculiar manner of union between the two, the hand can turn through nearly one hundred and eighty degrees. This, together with the ninety degrees of rotation possible in the shoulder joint, makes it possible to turn the hand almost two hundred and seventy degrees when the elbow is extended.

THE LIGAMENTS OF THE ELBOW JOINT

The ligaments are three in number, namely:
1. The articular capsule
2. The ulnar collateral ligament
3. The radial collateral ligament (Figs. 7 & 8)

THE ARTICULAR CAPSULE is attached to the front of the medial epicondyle and to the front of the humerus immediately above the coronoid and radial fossae, and below to the anterior surface of the coronoid process of the ulna. The posterior part is thin and membranous being attached above to the humerus and below it is fixed to the upper and lateral margins of the olecronon and to the posterior part of the annular ligament of the ulna behind the radial notch. It is also in relation behind with the tendon of the triceps brachii.

THE ULNAR COLLATERAL LIGAMENT is a thick, triangular band consisting of two portions, an anterior and a posterior, united by a thin, intermediate portion. THE ANTERIOR PORTION is directed obliquely forward and is attached above by its apex to the front part of the medial epicondyle of the humerus and below by its broad base to the medial margin of the coronoid process. THE POSTERIOR PORTION is also of triangular form, is attached above to the back part of the medial epicondyle, below to the medial margin of the olecranon. This ligament is in relation with the triceps brachii, the flexor carpi ulnaris and the ulnar nerve.

THE RADIAL COLLATERAL LIGAMENT is a short, narrow, fibrous band attached above to a depression below the lateral epicondyle of the humerus, below to the annular ligament, and is then inserted into the lateral margin of the ulna. It is intimately blended with the tendon of origin of the supinator.

The Nerve Supply of the elbow joint is as follows: A twig from the ulnar as it passes between the medial condyle and the olecronon, a filament from the musculocutaneous and two from the median nerve (Fig. 11).

THE MUSCLES OF THE ELBOW

The seven muscles which are associated with the elbow are as follows:

1. The biceps brachii
2. The brachialis
3. The triceps brachii
4. The brachioradialis
5. The pronator teres
6. The pronator quadratus
7. The supinator

The three first mentioned above have been described with the shoulder and arm on pages 34-37.

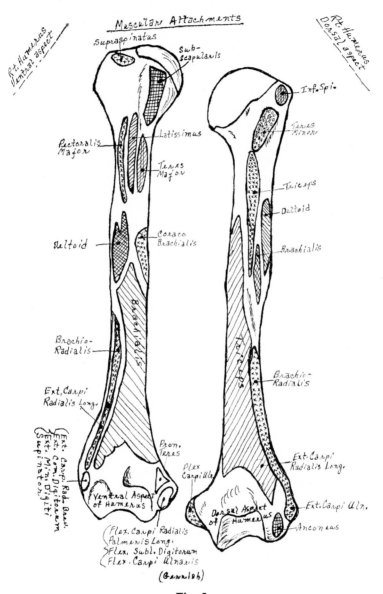

Muscular Attachments

Rt. Humerus
Ventral aspect

Supraspinatus

Sub-scapularis

Pectoralis Major

Latissimus

Teres Major

Deltoid

Coraco Brachialis

Brachialis

Brachio-Radialis

Ext. Carpi Radialis Long.

Ext. Carpi Rad. Brev.
Ext. Com. Digitorum
Ext. Min. Digiti
Supinator.

Pron. Teres

Ventral Aspect of Humerus

(Flex. Carpi Radialis
(Palmaris Long.
(Flex. Subl. Digitorum
(Flex. Carpi Ulnaris

Rt. Humerus
Dorsal aspect

Inf. Spi.

Teres Minor

Triceps

Deltoid

Brachialis

Triceps

Brachio-Radialis

Ext. Carpi Radialis Long.

Plex Carpilln

Dorsal Aspect of Humerus

Ext. Carpi Uln.

Anconeus

(Gennich)

Fig. 5

41

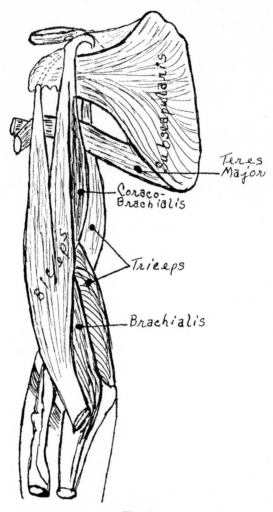

Fig. 6

MUSCLES OF RIGHT SHOULDER AND ARM
— Anterior View   (Gerrish)

THE BRACHIORADIALIS: *Origin:* It originates in the upper two-thirds of the external condyloid ridge of the humerus. *Insertion:* It inserts into the external surface of the radius at its lower end. *Structure:* Arising directly from the humerus, the fibers join the lower tendon in a penniform manner. *Action:* The position of the brachioradialis indicates that it is a flexor of the elbow; its leverage is long but its angle of pull very short. *Isolated action of the brachialis:* It flexes the elbow with great force and either pronates or supinates, according to the position of the hand when it contracts. *Nerve Supply:* This is from the fifth and sixth cervical nerves.

THE PRONATOR TERES: This is a small, spindle shaped muscle lying obliquely across the elbow in front and partly covered by the brachioradialis. *Origin:* It arises from the front side of the internal condyle of the humerus. *Insertion:* It inserts into the outer surface of the radius near its middle border. *Structure:* Fibers arising from the short tendons join the tendon of insertion obliquely, the latter lying beneath the muscle for half its length. *Action:* In flexion only, it acts with the biceps, its pronating action neutralizing some of the supinating action of the larger muscle. Otherwise it is a pronator. *Nerve Supply:* The median nerve.

THE PRONATOR QUADRATUS: This is a thin, square sheet of parallel fibers lying deep on the forearm near the wrist. *Origin:* It arises from the lower fourth of the front side of the ulna. *Insertion:* It inserts into the lower fourth of the front side of the radius. *Structure:* Parallel fibers attached directly to the bone. *Action:* The chief action is pronation. *Nerve Supply:* The volar interosseous.

THE SUPINATOR: This is a small muscle situated on the back of the arm just below the elbow. *Origin:* The external condyle of the humerus, the neighboring parts of the ulna and the ligaments in between. *Insertion:* The outer surface of the upper third of the radius. *Structure:* The muscle consists mainly of parallel fibers. *Action:* Supination as is indicated by its position. *Nerve Supply:* The posterior interosseous.

The Radio-Ulnar Articulations

The articulation of the radius with the ulna is effected by ligaments which connect the extremities as well as the body of these bones. The ligaments may be divided into three sets:

1. Those of the proximal radio-ulnar articulation

2. The middle radio-ulnar ligaments

3. The ligaments of the distal radio-ulnar articulation

THE PROXIMAL RADIO-ULNAR ARTICULATION or superior radio-ulnar joint is trochoid, a pivot joint between the circumference of the head of the radius and the ring formed by the radial notch of the ulna and the annular ligament. THE ANNULAR LIGAMENT is a strong band of fibers which encircles the head of the radius and retains it in contact with the radial notch of the ulna. It forms about four-fifths of the osseofibrous ring, and is attached to the anterior and posterior margins of the radial notch. Its upper border blends with the anterior and posterior ligaments of the elbow, while from its lower border a thin, loose membrane passes to be attached to the neck of the radius. Its deep surface is smooth and lined by synovial membrane which continues with the elbow joint.

Movements are limited to rotary ones of the head, or the radius within the ring formed by the annular ligament and the radial notch of the ulna. Pronation is forward rotation and supination is backward rotation. Pronation is performed by the pronator teres and pronator quadratus. Supination is done by the biceps brachii and the supinator assisted slightly by the extensor muscles of the thumb.

THE MIDDLE RADIO-ULNAR UNION: The shafts of the radius and ulna are connected by the oblique cord and the interosseous membrane. The oblique cord is a small, flattened band extending downward and lateralward from the lateral side of the tubercle of the ulna at the base of the coronoid process to the radius just a little below the radial tuberosity. Its fibers run in the opposite direction to those of the interosseous membrane.

THE INTEROSSEOUS MEMBRANE is a broad, thin plane of fibrous tissue descending obliquely downward and medialward from the interosseous crest of the radius to that of the ulna. The lower part of the membrane is attached to the posterior of the two lines into which the interosseous crest of the radius divides it. This

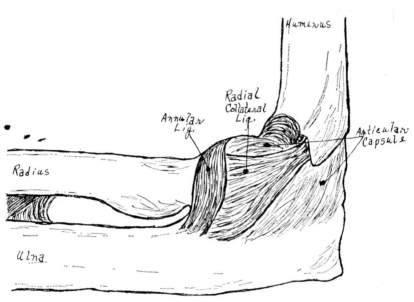

Fig. 7
LEFT ELBOW JOINT — Lateral Aspect   (Gray)

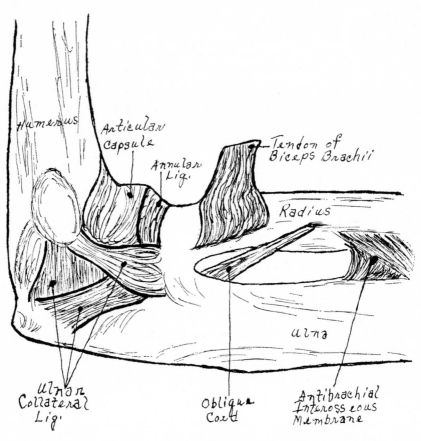

Fig. 8
LEFT ELBOW JOINT — Medial Aspect   (Gray)

46

membrane serves to connect the bones and to increase the extent of surface for the attachment of the deep muscles.

THE DISTAL RADIO-ULNAR ARTICULATION is a pivot joint formed between the head of the ulna and the ulnar notch on the lower end of the radius. The articular surfaces are connected by the following ligaments:

1. THE VOLAR RADIO-ULNAR LIGAMENT is a narrow band of fibers extending from the anterior margin to the ulnar notch of the radius to the front of the head of the ulna.

2. THE DORSAL RADIO-ULNAR LIGAMENT extends between corresponding surfaces of the dorsal aspect of the articulation.

3. THE ARTICULAR DISC is triangular in shape and is placed transversely beneath the head of the ulna, binding the lower ends of the ulna and radius firmly together. Its periphery is thicker than its center, which is occasionally perforated. It is attached by its apex to a depression between the styloid process and the head of ulna and by its base to the prominent edge of the radius which separates the ulnar notch from the carpal articular surface. Its margins are united to the ligaments of the wrist joint.

THE RADIO-CARPAL ARTICULATION

The wrist joint is a condyloid articulation and the parts forming it are the lower end of the radius, the under surface of the articular disc above, and the navicular, lunate and triangular bones below. The articular surface of the radius and undersurface of the articular disc together form a transverse elliptical, concave surface, the receiving cavity. The superior articular surfaces of the navicular, lunate and triangular form a smooth, convex surface, the condyle of which is received into the concavity. The joint is surrounded by a capsule and strengthened by the following ligaments:

1. The volar radio-carpal
2. The dorsal radio-carpal
3. The ulnar collateral
4. The radial collateral

THE VOLAR RADIO-CARPAL ligament is a broad, membranous band attached above to the anterior margin of the lower end of the radius, to its styloid process and to the front of the lower end of the ulna. Its fibers pass downward and medialward to be inserted into the volar surface of the navicular, lunate and triangular bones, some fibers being continued to the capitate.

THE DORSAL RADIO-CARPAL LIGAMENT is less thick and strong than the volar and is attached above to the posterior border of the lower end of the radius. Its fibers are directed obliquely downward and medialward and are fixed below to the dorsal surfaces of the navicular, lunate and triangular bones. It is in relation behind with the extensor tendons of the fingers, in front it is blended with the articular disc.

THE ULNAR COLLATERAL LIGAMENT is a rounded cord, attached above to the end of the styloid process of the ulna, dividing below into two fasciculae, one of which is attached to the medial side of the triangular bone and the other to the pisiform bone and the transverse carpal ligament.

THE RADIAL COLLATERAL LIGAMENT extends from the tip of the styloid process of the radius to the radial side of the navicular, some of its fibers becoming attached to the greater multangular bone and the transverse carpal ligament. It is in relation with the radial artery which separates the ligaments from the tendons of the abductor pollicis longus and extensor brevis.

Chapter IV

THE WRIST AND HAND

THE INTERCARPAL ARTICULATIONS

The intercarpal articulations may be subdivided into three sets, namely:

1. The articulations of the proximal row of carpal bones.
2. The articulations of the distal row of carpal bones.
3. The articulations of the two rows with each other.

THE ARTICULATIONS OF THE PROXIMAL ROW OF CARPAL BONES are arthrodial joints. The navicular, lunate and triangular are connected by the dorsal, volar and interosseous ligaments.

THE ARTICULATIONS OF THE DISTAL ROW OF CARPAL BONES are also arthrodial joints, the bones being connected to the dorsal, volar and interosseous ligaments.

THE ARTICULATIONS OF THE TWO ROWS OF CARPAL BONES WITH EACH OTHER. The joints between the navicular, lunate and triangular bones on the one hand, and the second row of carpal bones on the other is named the midcarpal joint and is made up of three different portions. In the center, the head of the capitate and the superior surface of the hamate articulate with the deep, cup-shaped cavity formed by the navicular and lunate bones. This constitutes a sort of ball and socket joint. On the radial side, the greater and lesser multangulars articulate with the navicular. On the ulnar side, the hamate articulates with the triangular forming gliding joints.

THE LIGAMENTS OF THE INTERCARPAL ARTICULATIONS are as follows:

1. The volar
2. The dorsal
3. The ulnar
4. The radial collateral

The synovial membrane is very extensive and bounds a synovial cavity of very irregular shape.

MOVEMENTS OF THE WRIST

The articulation of the hand and wrist, considered as a whole, involves four articular surfaces, namely:

1. The inferior surface of the radius and the articular disc.

2. The superior surfaces of the navicular, lunate and triangular, the pisiform having no essential part in the movements of the hand.

3. The "S" shaped surface formed by the inferior surfaces of the navicular, lunate and triangular.

4. The reciprocal surfaces formed by the upper surfaces of the bones of the second row.

These four surfaces form two joints:

A. The proximal — the wrist joint proper.
B. The distal — the mid-carpal joint.

THE WRIST JOINT PROPER is a true condyloid articulation, therefore all movements by rotation are permitted and flexion and extension are most free. Of these two, a greater amount of extension than flexion is allowed because the articular surfaces extend farther on the dorsal than on the volar surface of the carpal bones. In this movement the carpal bones rotate on a transverse axis drawn between the tips of the styloid process of the radius, and the ulna. A certain amount of adduction (or ulnar flexion) and abduction (radial flexion) is also permitted. The former is considerably greater in extent than the latter on account of the shortness of the styloid process of the ulna, abduction being soon limited by the contact of the styloid process of the radius with the greater multangular. In this movement, the carpus revolves upon an anteroposterior axis drawn through the center of the wrist. Finally, circumduction is permitted by the combined and consecutive movements of adduction, extension, abduction and flexion. No rotation is possible but the effect of rotation is obtained by the pronation and supination of the radius and ulna.

THE DISTAL OR MID-CARPAL JOINT: The chief movements permitted in the midcarpal joint are flexion and extension, plus a slight amount of rotation. In flexion and extension, which are the movements most freely enjoyed, the greater and lesser multangulars on the radial side and the hamate on the ulnar side, glide forward and backward on the navicular and triangular respectively, while the head of the capitate and the superior surface of the hamate rotate in the cup-shaped cavity of the navicular and hamate. Flexion in the joint is freer than extension and there also is a trifling amount of rotation. A very small amount of rotation is also permitted when the head of the capitate rotates around a vertical axis drawn through its own center while at the same time a slight, gliding movement takes place in the lateral and medial portions of the joint.

THE CARPO-METACARPAL ARTICULATION OF THE THUMB

This joint is a reciprocal reception between the first metacarpal and the greater multangular. It enjoys great freedom of movement on account of the configuration of its articular surface, which is saddle shaped. The joint is surrounded by a capsule which is thick but loose and passes from the circumference of the base of the metacarpal bone to the rough edge bounding the articular surfaces of the greater multangular. It is thickest laterally and dorsally and is lined by synovial membrane.

MOVEMENTS OF THE THUMB: In this articulation, the movements permitted are flexion and extension in the plane of the palm of the hand; abduction and adduction in a plane at right angles to the palm and also circumduction and apposition. It is by the movement of apposition that the tip of the thumb is brought into contact with the volar surfaces of the slightly flexed fingers. This movement is effected through the medium of a small, sloping facet on the anterior lip of the saddle shaped articular surface of the greater multangular. The flexor muscles pull the corresponding part of the articular surface of the metacarpal bone on this facet, and the movement of apposition is then carried out by the adductors.

ARTICULATIONS OF THE OTHER FOUR METACARPAL BONES WITH THE CARPUS

The joints between the carpus and the second, third, fourth and fifth metacarpal bones are arthrodial. The bones are united by dorsal, volar and interosseous ligaments. *Movements:* The movements permitted in the carpo-metacarpal articulations of the fingers are limited to a slight gliding of the articular surfaces upon each other, the extent of which varies in the different joints. The metacarpal bone of the little finger is more movable than that of the ring finger. The metacarpals of the index and middle fingers are the least movable.

51

THE INTERMEDIATE CARPAL ARTICULATIONS

The bases of the second, third, fourth and fifth metacarpal bones articulate with one another by small surfaces covered with cartilage and are connected together by the dorsal, volar and interosseous ligaments.

THE METACARPAL-PHALANGEAL ARTICULATIONS

The metacarpal-phalangeal articulations are of the condyloid kind, formed by the reception of the rounded heads of the metacarpal bones into shallow cavities on the proximal ends of the first phalanges, with one exception, the thumb, which presents more of the characteristics of a ginglymus joint. Each articulation has one volar and two collateral ligaments. The dorsal surfaces of these joints are covered by the expansions of the extensor tendons, together with some loose areolar tissue which connects the deep surfaces of the tendons to the bones. *Movements:* The movements which occur in these articulations are flexion, extension, adduction, abduction and circumduction. The movements of abduction and adduction are limited and cannot be performed with the fingers flexed.

THE ARTICULATIONS OF THE DIGITS

The interphalangeal articulations are hinge joints and each has one volar and two collateral ligaments. The arrangement of these ligaments is similar to those in the metacarpo-phalangeal articulations. The extensor tendons take the place of the posterior ligaments (Fig. 9). *Movements:* The only movements permitted in the interphalangeal joints are flexion and extension. These movements are more extensive between the first and second phalanges than between the second and third. The amount of flexion is very considerable, but extension is limited by the volar and volar collateral ligaments.

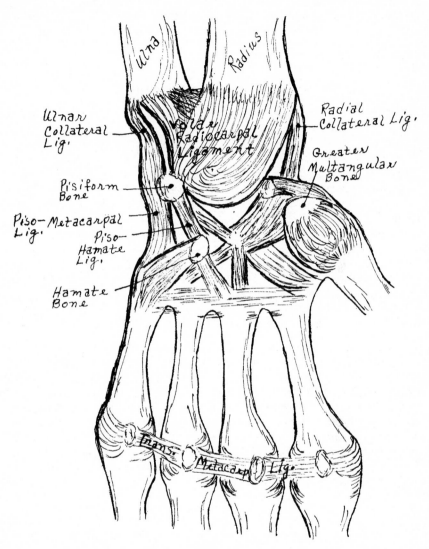

Fig. 9

LIGAMENTS OF LEFT WRIST AND METACARPUS
Volar Aspect   (Gray)

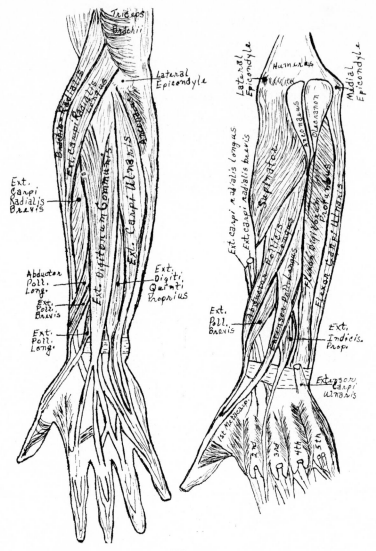

Fig. 10

Post. Surface of Forearm   Post. Surface of Forearm
Superficial Muscles   Deep Muscles

(Gray)

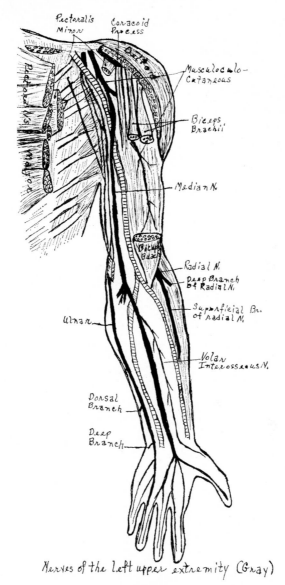

Nerves of the left upper extremity (Gray)

Fig. 11

55

Chapter V

PAIN IN THE SHOULDER, ARM AND HAND

Pain is usually the first symptom to present itself and sometimes it is the only one. The complete syndrome can include sensory and motor changes caused by interference with the central or peripheral nervous systems with involvement of the sympathetic nerves. Vascular disturbances may also be in evidence.

Since pain alone can be indicative of shoulder derangement, it is therefore the most important symptom and arises from subluxations of the bony articulations or a derangement of any component of the whole area. There are patterns that indicate specific disorders, most of which localize the pain to the shoulder and neck area. The pain may be in the shoulder joint only, or in the joint in conjunction with radiating pains. These discomforts have a multiplicity of origins and may be described by the patient as pressure, stretching, cutting, gnawing, cramping or combinations of these, all adding up to great misery to the sufferer.

The pain mechanism can usually be classified into three categories:

1. Those with the dominant pain in the shoulder and neck.
2. Those with the dominant pain in the shoulder only.
3. Those in which the shoulder is painful and combined with radiating pains.

Not all shoulder conditions will follow this pattern but the vast majority will do so.

THE CAUSES OF PAIN IN THE NECK AND SHOULDER REGION

The causes are: local disorders such as postural and occupational strain; subluxations; fibrositis; muscular sprains and tears or soft tissue derangements. Reflex pain to the area from more distant parts, such as the head, chest and abdomen, are not uncommon. Since this is a frequent occurrence, it is well to bear this point in mind when examining the patient who presents neck and shoulder discomfort.

56

The area at the base of the skull, the back of the neck and the root of the neck contain the attachments of the muscles, some of which are the powerful suspensory ones, and the duties of these muscles are to support and balance the head and suspend the shoulders. This is an involuntary function.

Pain in the shoulder and neck may further be caused by sinusitis, migraine or emotional tension. These conditions, when combined with anatomical derangements in this area, causes a vicious circle, each making the other worse.

ARTICULAR PAIN: Major nerve trunks passing a joint supply sensory branches to it, to the periarticular structures, the periosteum, tendon insertions and the ligamentous attachments. These structures are freely ennervated and are particularly susceptible to stretch and strain stimuli and will create pain of greater intensity than the postural type causing nerve pressure. Therefore, some definitely abnormal movement is required to cause the sprains and subluxations, usually the violent type of accidents, such as falls with the arm extended or some such similar happening. Pain through this channel is localized to the joint area. When the capsule or synovium are injured, the pain is more diffuse and not distinctly related to the joint.

RADIATING PAINS: The sharp, shooting and irregular pain from the shoulder to the base of the thumb or fingers is due to nerve root pressure and is caused by cervical disc involvement. The sensory root supplies an area of skin or dermatome, and also a group of deep structures namely, muscles, tendons and bone. The nerve roots most frequently involved are the sixth and seventh cervicals and much of the sensation of the shoulder musculature is derived from the sixth cervical. The skin distribution of the same root is along the forearm to the base of the thumb. This is one explanation of the deep shoulder discomfort felt in such lesions.

RADIATING PAIN OF VASCULAR ORIGIN: There is another form of radiating pain which is predominantly more vascular than nervous in origin. The great vessels may be affected either by compression or traction or both, thereby causing many disorders and pain. The source of such difficulties lie in the shoulder girdle and first rib area, but the discomforting pains are felt in the hands and fingers. The usual symptoms are aching, a feeling of fullness in the fingers, tingling of the fingertips followed by numbness, stiffness and weakness in the fingers and hand. These symptoms result from arterial and venous pressure.

The recognition of the type of pain and understanding its cause is most important. The principal symptoms are an aching pain in the shoulder, arm and forearm with a feeling of numbness in the fingers and entire hand. The hand may feel limp and this may be followed by a biting or prickly sensation. The main cause has been laid to irritation and pressure on the vascular bundle and this leads to the peripheral changes.

The writer has elaborated more on this syndrome and explained the cause and correction under the scalene anticus syndrome in the following chapter.

Chapter VI

THE SCALENE TRIANGLE

THE ABNORMAL SCALENE TRIANGLE PLUS ITS COMPONENT PARTS EQUALS THE SHOULDER, ARM AND HAND SYNDROME

The component parts of the scalene triangle consist of the scalenus anticus muscle at the front, the scalenus medius and the scalenus posticus at the rear, and at times the latter two are blended into one. The first rib completes the triangle and forms its base. The brachial plexus and the subclavian artery are contained within the space between the anticus and medius muscles while the subclavian vein lies in front of the scalenus anticus in a space between the first rib and the clavicle. From a chiropractic viewpoint it is readily apparent that compression and pressure in this area could result in many varied symptoms relating to the shoulder, arm and hand syndrome (Figs. 12 and 13).

Far too little attention has been given to these relatively small and seemingly unimportant muscles. Gray's anatomy lists them as the lateral vertebral muscles, and their action is, from above, to elevate the first and second ribs and therefore they are considered inspiratory muscles. Acting from below they bend the vertebral column to one side or the other, and if the muscles on both sides act simultaneously, the vertebral column is slightly flexed.

THE SCALENUS ANTICUS: It lies deeply at the side of the neck behind the sternocleidomastoid muscle. It arises from the anterior tubercles of the transverse processes of the third, fourth, fifth and sixth cervical vertebrae and, descending almost vertically, is inserted by a narrow, flat tendon into the scalene tubercle on the inner border of the first rib and into the ridge on the upper surface of the rib in front of the subclavian groove.

THE SCALENUS MEDIUS: It is the largest and the longest of the three scalene muscles and arises from the posterior tubercles of the transverse processes of the lower six cervical vertebrae. It descends along the side of the vertebral column and is inserted by a broad attachment into the upper surface of the first rib between the tubercle and the subclavian groove.

THE SCALENUS POSTICUS: It is the smallest and most deeply seated of the three scaleni and arises by two or three separate tendons from the posterior tubercles of the transverse processes of the lower two or three cervical vertebrae and is inserted by a thin tendon into the outer surface of the second rib behind the attachment of the serratus anterior. It is occasionally blended with the scalenus medius. The nerve supply of the scalene muscles comes from branches of the second to seventh cervical nerves.

The writer has found no common denominator in caring for the many and varying shoulder conditions. If one could name an area as the most important and most frequently involved in the greatest number of shoulder syndromes, it would be the area of the spine that makes up the brachial plexus. It will be shown how the scalene triangle has its effect upon this important region. It has been pointed out that the anterior scalene muscle arises from the transverse processes of the third, fourth, fifth and sixth cervical vertebrae and cruises downward to be inserted on the scalene tubercle at the upper, inner surface of the first rib. At each level from the fourth to the seventh cervical vertebrae, a branch is supplied to ennervate the muscles.

The picture that these muscles present is somewhat like an Indian tepee cut in half from top to bottom with the first rib acting as the floor, forming a triangle that is not quite geometrically perfect.

The scalenus anticus is attached in front of and slightly farther out on the rib than the scalenus medius, which is the largest of the three muscles. It forms the back of the triangle and is attached farther inward toward the cervical spine. The scalenus posticus is relatively small, and many times it is blended with the medius and is attached to the second rib. It does not have a direct effect on the so-called scalenus anticus syndrome.

The brachial plexus and the subclavian artery lie within this triangle between the anterior and medial scalene muscles. Therefore, any abnormal contracture of these muscles, such as irritation, spasm, short or hypertrophied muscles and similar aggravations will cause a contracture of the triangle. This results in a scissors-like or pincer-like action on the brachial plexus and the subclavian artery, and pressure is also put upon the subclavian vein which lies in front of the muscle in the space between the first rib and clavicle. Though this condition is usually known as the scalenus anticus syndrome, it is this writer's opinion that more than the scalenus anticus is at fault. In fact, the scalenus medius is also involved, and these two muscles, because of their attach-

60

ment to the first rib, will, when they contract, cause a superior subluxation of the first rib. This in turn produces compression and irritation to the brachial plexus and subclavian vessels because of their location above the first rib. Since the symptoms so produced are similar to those caused by a cervical rib, it is always advisable to use an x-ray examination in order to eliminate this abnormal growth as a causative factor.

There are other findings which necessitate a careful differential diagnosis. The pain of the scalenus anticus syndrome is similar to that encountered in a herniated disc, a thin disc or a subluxated vertebra, and again, the x-ray film becomes a most useful tool in establishing or eliminating these possibilities. The symptoms are many and varied. There may be pain in the shoulder girdle, arm, hand and chest which is similar to the pain in coronary artery disease or other forms of interthoracic pathology. It may cause pain and discomfort in the cervical region and upper or lower chest, or it may center in the scapular area and resemble the pain of gallbladder disease or phrenic nerve irritation. Most generally there is occipital pain and tenderness and often there is a sensation of heaviness or weight in the entire arm. The patient may complain of cold hands or fingers and numbness may be a frequent symptom. In mild cases there may be little or no pain, only a sensation of heaviness, at times associated with paresthesia affecting the ulnar or radial portions of the arm and hand. Occupations in which the arms are used a great deal, or those that require long periods of arm elevation may be a cause. There may be a suspicion of heart pain when the affected scalene lesion is on the left side, and when it is on the right, it is not infrequently diagnosed as pleurisy.

SUBCLAVIAN ARTERY PRESSURE

A spastic, hypertrophied scalenus may cause a narrowing of the acute angle formed by the anticus and medius and the first rib. The subclavian artery lies within this angle, and when compressed may cause severe pain in the upper portions of the arm and hand, and the fingers may be cooler than those on the unaffected side. There may also be a sensation of a dull, heavy arm, as though a weight had been placed on it. Other complaints frequently mentioned by the patient can include a severe cramp-like ache with a sensation of numbness and tingling, and the handclasp will usually be weak.

SUBCLAVIAN VEIN PRESSURE

Compression of the subclavian vein is not usually directly produced by a spastic scalene muscle. Rather, it comes about because the spastic muscles, by their pull, raise the first rib, thereby narrowing the costo-clavicular space which in turn causes the direct venous pressure.

This small anatomical region presents only one of the many facets in the shoulder, and related area syndromes. However, it is most important from a chiropractic viewpoint since it presents five distinct locations of frequent nerve pressure and irritation with possible vascular compression.

1. Subluxations of the cervical vertebrae which affect the nerves supplying the scalene muscles (second to seventh cervical nerves) thereby causing irritation and shortening of the muscles.

2. Subluxations of the vertebrae affecting the brachial plexus.

3. Subluxation of the first rib and its subsequent effects on the brachial plexus, the subclavian artery and vein.

4. The pincer-like action by the scalene muscles directly upon the brachial plexus and the subclavian artery.

5. The area of the first rib and clavicle which is the point of compression when the costo-clavicular space is narrowed, and this also affects the subclavian vein.

Further elaboration is needed to clarify the many ramifications and pathways of direct pain, reflex pain and discomfort that this abnormal condition can cause.

BRACHIAL PLEXUS PRESSURE

Let us review the brachial plexus and its relationship to the triangular aperture. The brachial plexus is formed by the intricate interlacement of the anterior primary division of the four cervical nerves mentioned above, and the first dorsal or thoracic nerves, also receiving contributions from the second, and third thoracic, occasionally also from the fourth. After leaving the intervertebral foramina, these nerves converge toward the upper surface of the first rib and then emerge in the space between the scalenus anticus and the scalenus medius muscles. From the side of the neck they then pass beneath the clavicle and enter the axilla through the apex.

There are several diagnostic signs which suggest the presence of this syndrome, namely:

1. The disorder is ushered in by neck and shoulder discomfort with pain in the upper arm, hand and fingers.

2. The pain may have a vague, aching quality and the patient has difficulty in outlining the exact zone. This is in contrast to cervical root pressure and peripheral nerve lesions or the pain caused by a cervical rib.

3. There is fullness in the suprascapular space.

4. There is tenderness of the scalene muscles on the affected side.

5. Extension of the neck increases the pain, flexion has a tendency to relieve it. In some cases chest movement is irritating.

6. A significant test is the effect of pressure on the scalenus anticus with the finger. Place the middle finger one inch above the clavicle in the posterior area of the sternocleidomastoideus. Push the finger toward the spine. The resistance thus encountered is the scalenus anticus. Compression causes intensified pain and distress when compared with the same pressure on the unaffected side. This test is performed by tilting the patient's head back and away from the tender side (Fig. 12).

7. If tilting the head toward the painful side with downward pressure causes increased pain and a radiation of it, and if stretching or extending the neck causes complete or partial relief from it when sufficient force is exerted, then the cause may be assumed to be a vertebral or disc lesion rather than extra-vertebral. If, on the other hand, the cause of the pain were in the scalene muscles, then compression of the scaleni would relax the muscles and ease the pain (Figs. 15, 16, 17).

8. If the motion of the shoulder is restricted, it is a local lesion in the shoulder girdle and we do not have a primary scalene syndrome.

The Doctors Judovitch and Bates, in their extensive research on the scalenus anticus syndrome, find that there are two types, namely the primary and secondary. Quoting from their book, "Pain Syndromes," they say: "A primary scalene syndrome is one in which the symptoms originate in and are due to an intrinsic disturbance of the anterior scalene muscles, spasm, hypertrophy or myositis usually due to trauma. This may be due to acute injury directly affecting the muscles or it may be chronic in the form of postural defects or occupational strain or developmental variations."

"The secondary scalene syndrome may be defined as one in which the symptoms are due to reflex spasm of the anterior scalene muscles causing irritation of the structures in the shoulder girdle or by disturbances of the segments which ennervate these structures. Among the lesions which may cause reflex scalene spasm are interspinal spacetaking and inflammatory lesion of the cervical spine; radiculitis of the fourth to seventh cervical nerve roots; malignancy of the cervical spine; disease, trauma or inflammatory lesions of the skeletal structures supplied by the fourth to seventh cervical segments, including the central diaphragm and probably the pericardium. Interesting phenomena are the reflex scalene syndromes which may follow coronary thrombosis."

"A scalene syndrome, herniated disc or other root irritating lesion may cause pain in the chest and arm which simulates coronary disease. On the other hand, it appears that the scalene spasm may follow myocardial infarction, the muscles become full and tight; pressure causes reproduction and radiation of the pain. This is not uncommon in persistence of pain following an infarction. Clinically, this condition has none of the characteristics of the shoulder-hand syndrome."

These authors explain further as follows: "When a myocardial infarct develops, a resultant pericardial irritation may affect the sensory ending of the phrenic nerve. This in turn causes an intrasegmental reflex reference of pain in the sensory distribution of C3, C4, and C5 segments, causing pain which is referred to the neck and shoulder girdle. If the stimuli are adequate, a spasm of the anterior scalene muscle develops and a sensory motor reflex."

"It is extremely important that the two types be distinguished by clinical methods before attempting surgical procedures. The primary type will obtain complete relief with procaine injection and surgery, but the secondary, or reflex type will obtain only partial relief. Yet, the signs and symptoms presented by each may, in certain instances, be identical."

Dr. Bateman, in his book, "The Shoulder and Environs," states: "Neurovascular disorder in the absence of a cervical rib, has long been ascribed to a tight scalenus anticus muscle. A short, hypertrophied muscle can compress subclavian vessels and lower nerve trunk, resulting in significant symptoms almost identical with those of a cervical rib. There has been a tendency to lump many disorders under this heading, which accounts for some of the unsatisfactory results of scaleneotomy. The syndrome does occur, but it should be appreciated that there are specific signs and symptoms which separate the true scalene compression from other causes of radiating discomfort."

There can be no doubt that these muscles become tight, short, constricting bands and do cause pressure, compression and irritation on the nerves and subclavian vessels. It is obvious that this area should be thoroughly investigated from a chiropractic viewpoint. We have long known the effect of nerve pressure caused by spinal subluxations and the dramatic recoveries that have occurred when the nerve pressures were normalized.

The shoulder syndrome and its many causes has long been of interest to the writer, and through the experience of many years, he is convinced that this is an important area to be dealt with in the difficult shoulder cases. It is most interesting to note the reflex action of the scalene muscles following myocardial disorders, also the explanation given by Judovich and Bates. We, as doctors of chiropractic, ought to investigate as to whether the reflex action of the scalene muscles working in reverse could be a cause in coronary and other myocardial diseases.

From the research done by the three eminent authorities quoted, it appears that they agree that surgery is not the entire answer. They advise corrective postural exercises, changes in sleeping habits, rest, a change in occupation and they also strongly advise traction. They use such terms as herniated discs, thinning of the discs, disc protrusion, interspinal spacetaking, disturbances of the segments which ennervate the structures, and they give them as reasons for the reflex scalene spasm. While this is excellent terminology, it is interesting to note that the word subluxation is not mentioned, neither is the common and much overused diagnosis of slipped disc.

Dr. Bateman also states: "By far the majority of cervical disc protrusions recover on conservative treatment and operation is rarely needed." He further states under the heading of "Conservative Treatment" as follows: "The principle is to release the pressure of the disc on the cervical root and this is best accomplished by traction. The simplest method is to provide the patient with his own traction apparatus. It is important to use a flat, firm bed and preferably with a bolster pillow which fits snugly in the nape of the neck. Most cases respond to this program but there remain some to whom it is necessary to apply a molded cervical collar."

The most important factor in the production of the scalene syndrome is trauma. This may be any injury directly affecting the muscles or it may be chronic, caused by occupational strain, poor postural habits or developmental variations. These lesions, in the writer's opinion, cause subluxations of the cervical region. The subluxations may at first be minor, affecting the branches from the second to seventh cervical nerves which supply these muscles. This causes irritaton and tension in the scalene group.

Since we have covered the origin and insertion of the three scaleni, we can see that these muscles, because of their positioning, act as guy wires upon the cervical area with the first rib as the point of anchorage. Any shortening of these muscles will cause a downward pull on the vertebrae producing a pincer-like effect on the intervertebral cartilages and consequently also a thinning of the disc, more nerve pressure with added irritation and tension of the muscles thereby causing a scissors-like action on the brachial nerve and artery which lie between the scalene anticus and medius muscles. As the pull of the shortened and constricted muscles becomes greater, the first rib gives way and is subluxated upward which in turn closes the triangular space to a greater degree. Thus the space becomes more restricted and produces a sphincter like action upon the neurovascular bundle, and the subclavian vein is compressed in its course between the clavicle and the first rib. When this train of events takes place, the symptoms become severe and varied.

The question now is: "What can be done from a chiropractic standpoint?" First, of course, the subluxation in the cervical region must be adjusted. The chiropractic doctor need not be told how to do this. However, many times a well executed adjustment does not immediately normalize the shortened and tense scalene muscles and the pain and discomfort of the syndrome will still persist. The reason is that the leverage and pull of these muscles causes a loss of integrity and stability of the discs, thus allowing a questionable spacing of the spinal segments in the cervical region. In other words, the adjustment without case management does not give the complete and necessary correction because the action of the spasmed muscles is such as to produce recurring subluxations.

Proper case management is most important in caring for this type of lesion. Corrective exercises, occupational change or rest is to be advised during the period of treatment. Sleeping habits should be investigated and a firm, hard mattress advised. The patient should be told not to sleep face down with the head turned to one side. In some cases, two or three pillows should be recommended so that the patient's spine and head are supported beginning with the area of the tenth dorsal vertebra. Traction is of very great benefit and supervised intermittent traction in the doctor's office is the most effective. If that is not available, then the head halter type that the patient can use at home, should be substituted. Sometimes a cervical collar is beneficial.

The writer has found it to be true that the adjustment of the first rib is just as important as adjusting the offending cervical vertebrae in the management of this syndrome. Both must be corrected in order to give the patient quick and lasting results. The steps and reasons why the adjustment of the first rib is of such great importance in correcting this syndrome will be outlined here. The first rib gives the best leverage in releasing the tension of the scalene muscles. The contact on the first rib should be taken in the area of posterior lateral border of the sternocleidomastoid muscle, making the contact as close as possible to the scalene tubercle where the scalenus anticus inserts. This will be about one inch higher and approximately two and one-half inches posterior of the clavicle, depending upon the size and muscular development of the patient.

With a firm contact, take the slack out of the muscles. The superior rib is then adjusted downward with a fast, short thrust. The object is not only to adjust the superior rib subluxation downward, but also create a pulling stretch and quick release of the scalene muscles. This move, when executed properly, produces a beneficial reaction upon the vertebrae and discs. By using the first rib as leverage, a rippling force is exerted through the muscles and to the transverse processes of the lower six cervical vertebrae. This rippling effect occurs because of the method of attachment of the muscles to each transverse in the affected area and it could be described as similar to the effect of throwing a pebble into a still pool of water. The rippling effect cannot be obtained in a muscle such as the sternocleidomastoid because it is not attached to the individual transverse processes of the vertebrae. Tension and spasm of the scalene muscles should not be confused with torticollis. Even though the sternocleidomastoid is in close association with the scalene group, it is not necessarily involved. (First Rib Adjustment. Figs. 62, 63, 64.)

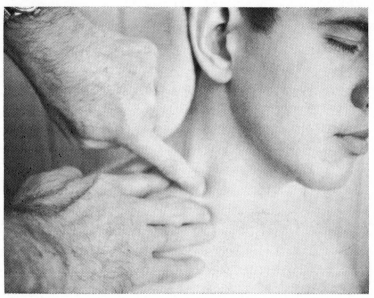

Fig. 12
Palpating for Tension and Tenderness in the Scalenus Anticus

Most of the time it is possible to palpate this area by forcing the finger into the side of the clavicular insertion of the sternocleidomastoideus and pushing it medially and downward while at the same time bringing the patient's head toward the painful side. This will relax the muscle. Then with the fingers straddling the sternocleidomastoid and the muscle forced medially, the patient's head is straightened and brought slightly to the opposite side. This brings the scalenus anticus forward so that in most cases it can be palpated. It will aid in palpation if the patient will take a deep breath and hold for a few seconds.

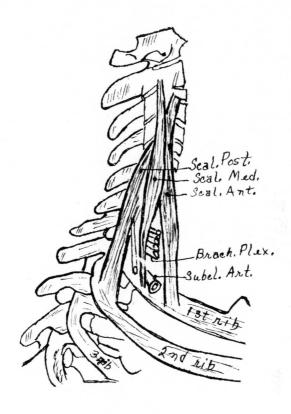

Fig. 13
THE SCALENI   (Gray)

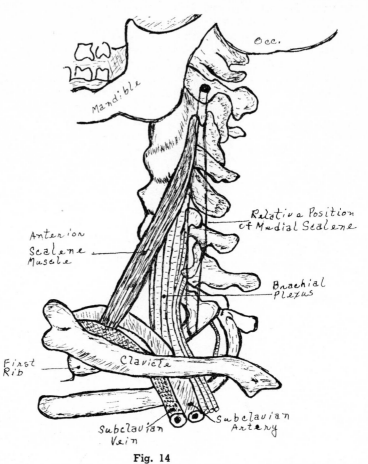

Fig. 14

Schematic Drawing Showing Relationship of Subclavian Artery and Vein, Brachial Plexus, Anterior and Medial Scalene Muscles

TESTING METHODS

The following 3 photographs, Figs. 15 to 17 inclusive, show the various ways of using traction and compression. The use of these tests is of significant importance in differentiating disc lesions from those of extra-vertebral soft tissues. If downward compression of the cervical spine intensifies discomfort and causes radiating pain, then, in most cases, the origin is from a disc lesion rather than from extra-vertebral involvement since it is reasonable to assume that downward muscular pressure would relax them somewhat and ease the discomfort. Conversely, when the lesion is in the extra-vertebral soft tissues, the use of traction can be expected to increase pain. Both types of lesions benefit a great deal from the use of traction, particularly the intermittent form.

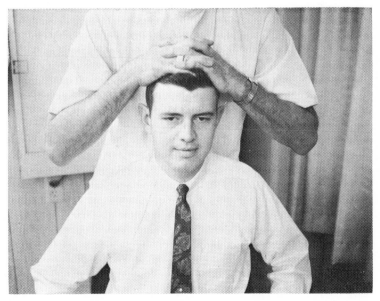

Fig. 15

The above picture shows the use of very firm pressure directly downward on the patient's head. If this causes an increase in pain, the cause of the difficulty is most often a disc lesion.

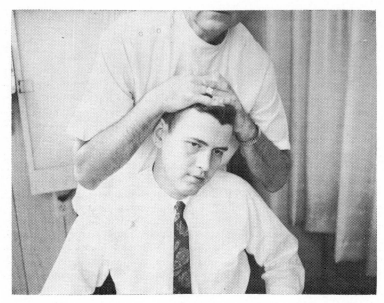

Fig. 16

In this test, the head is tilted toward the painful side and at the same time firm downward pressure is used. If the traction test shown in Fig. 17 has been used and found to give relief and the above test found to increase pain, it is almost invariably indicative of a disc lesion.

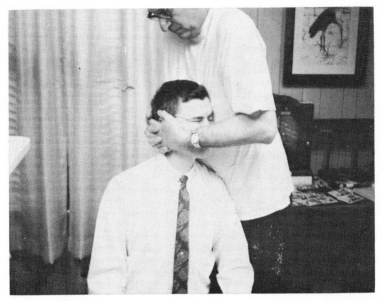

Fig. 17

The above picture shows a method of testing the effect of traction. The doctor locks his hands as shown on the affected side, steadies the other side of the patient's head against his own body and pulls straight up gradually but firmly. He then holds the traction for about 30 seconds and releases gradually. This test can also be done with the patient lying on his back on the adjusting table in which case an occipital-mandibular contact is taken. If traction eases the patient's discomfort, then the lesion is usually in the extravertebral soft tissues.

Occupations that require an individual to stand, and at the same time use the arms at shoulder height or above, put a great deal of stress and strain upon the entire shoulder structure and therefore the shoulder bursae frequently show pathological changes. The subacromial, sometimes called the subdeltoid, is the bursa most frequently affected. Differences in its size, thickness and position are not uncommon. It is located under the acromion process, on the superior portion of the humerus and is an extensive and important structure, complicated with extensions beneath the coracoid process and adjacent muscles.

The sole purpose of the subacromial bursa is to enhance the range of shoulder movements. It acts as a second joint for the head of the humerus and provides a lubricating system. Movement in front, at, and above shoulder level is made possible by this gliding mechanism. It allows the head of the humerus to roll under the arch and rotate on its long axis. The bursa is hung from the under side of the acromion, the coracoacromial ligament and the undersurface of the deltoid muscle. It extends under the coracoid process and over the subscapularis muscle, also under the muscles attached to the coracoid process. Its lower portion covers most of the greater tuberosity and extends medially over the rotator cuff.

Normally, the bursa is approximately one-fourth inch in depth and does not communicate with the shoulder joint, and its floor is the rotator cuff. Its location and function make it vulnerable to overstrain and wear and tear damage. The function of the bursa is to cushion the tuberosity from impinging on the arch so that minute irregularities and irritants are buffered by its presence (Figs. 18 and 19).

The bursa has a smooth, glistening inner surface which glides freely, and normally it does not contain a demonstrable amount of fluid. The deep layer of the bursa is closely adherent to the rotator cuff tendons while the superficial layer is adherent to the under surface of the acromion. When the walls of the bursa are inflamed or adherent to each other, the movement of the humerus is restricted (Figs. 18 and 19).

Inflammation is usually secondary following strain, overuse or injury, such as disorders involving the muscles and tendons which form the musculo-tendinous cuff, or injury to the bicipital mechanism.

Ordinarily, any common ailment characterized by pain which occurs around the shoulder joint, is labeled bursitis. There are a

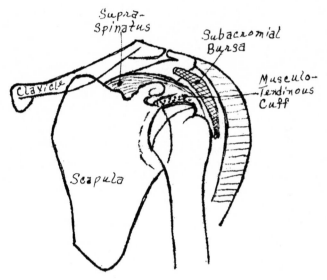

Fig. 18
Relations of the Subacromial Bursa

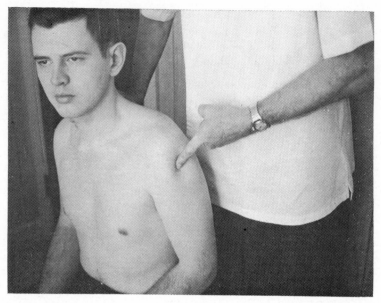

Fig. 19

This shows area of maximum tenderness in cases of subacromial bursitis, also called subdeltoid bursitis.

number of causes for this condition; accidental injuries by falls, repeated minor trauma from occupation or the performance of unaccustomed work, particularly overhead work. Since the bursa acts as a second joint, it is easy for it to become inflamed because of the extra duties thrown upon it.

In our specialized age of assembly line production, a person may be required to work with the hands and arms in a rather constant position, using the hands, arms and shoulders while repeatedly performing the same task. This kind of chronic overwork and strain can, in time, produce the shoulder symptom known as bursitis.

The writer has noticed in his own office that every spring and fall there would be an influx of patients with bursitis and tendinitis. Very often the patient would first blame the changeable weather for the pain, but when it did not disappear, would come in wondering what was wrong. With no history of accidental injury, it was simple to deduce that unaccustomed work was the culprit. In the cases of females, painting or wallpaper scraping in particular were the most frequent causes while with men it was generally pitching heavy grain bundles, scooping or throwing. In many cases, these patients showed a combination of tendinitis and bursitis.

In the treatment of bursitis we must first consider the nerve supply of the muscles, the tendinous cuff, and the bursa. Therefore, the cervical region is most important, particularly the adjustment of the first rib (Figs. 62 and 63), the supraspinatous (Figs. 92, 93 and 94), the infraspinatous (Figs. 95, 96, 97 and 98), as well as the adjustment of the cervical and upper dorsal area. The arm itself should never be manipulated since this will only irritate the situation. Case management is extremely important and in the great majority of cases the arm should be immobilized by taping as shown in Figs. 49, 50, 51 and 52, and then be placed in a sling since its weight alone, even without movement, can, and usually does, act as an irritant.

Most authorities agree that bursitis is a secondary condition, and this is no doubt true in the majority of cases where there is a history of trauma or occupational strain. Such situations will first involve the musculo-tendinous cuff and finally the bursa, which has had an additional strain placed upon it.

The writer believes that in some instances, particularly like those of the housewife who decides to remove the paper from the walls, that the bursa alone is seriously involved. Such persons will go to bed very tired but pain free, and will awaken in the night or

77

the next morning unable to move the arm and also be in intense pain. The area of pain, upon palpation, will be located on the sub-acromial (subdeltoid) bursa. This can be pinpointed by pressing on the medial portion of the deltoid muscle as shown in Fig. 19. Through the use of the adjustment and immobilization methods as outlined, the pain will subside and the arm return to normal within seven to ten days. The supportive measures will usually control the pain sufficiently so that the patient can sleep the first night after application, but there will be pain on movement.

The secondary type of bursitis involves the musculotendinous cuff and the bicipital tendon and is a more complicated condition. The case history will usually reveal previous injury or occupational strain or trauma. The patient generally is of middle age or older and these cases do not, as a rule, appear to have developed their symptoms overnight. The pain and discomfort in movement usually appears gradually while performing routine duties, or may creep up insidiously after an apparently negligible injury, perhaps a minor fall. The pain becomes progressively worse and the patient will come to the office when he cannot sleep because of it and is unable to raise his arm normally. He will usually hold it against his body, and even give it added support with the other hand.

In this situation the supportive measures to be used are the same as previously outlined but the treatment and recovery time will be longer than in the acute condition, and, when partial healing has taken place, the patient must be persuaded to do certain exercises that will be outlined at a later point. (See chapter on exercises.)

INJURIES TO THE MUSCULO-TENDINOUS CUFF

The four short rotator muscles of the shoulder, namely the supraspinatous, infraspinatous, teres minor and subscapularis, surround the joint on three sides, the inferior aspect being uncovered. These muscles constitute a very important muscular system and contribute to vital movements. The tendons of these muscles are inserted partly into the tuberosities of the humerus, the sulcus between the tuberosities and the articular surface. They are joined to the capsule so intimately that they can only be separated by cutting the cojoined tendons and capsule.

THE SUPERIOR PORTION OF THE CUFF is formed by the supraspinatous. It applies tension through a short lever on the top of the humerus and, as the muscle contracts, it pulls the head of the humerus directly into the socket in order to prevent upward displacement, which the deltoid tends to produce. In this way the action of force of the longer lever, the deltoid, is stabilized and allows this powerful muscle to act efficiently.

THE POSTERIOR PORTION OF THE CUFF is largely controlled by the infraspinatous with some contribution from the teres minor and both of these muscles have identical action. The infraspinatous is larger and bulkier than the supraspinatous and exerts a much stronger pull. The fleshy fibers extend well up into the capsule and its line of pull is downward and it externally rotates the humerus. It also acts as an extensor because of its insertion into the posterior part of the greater tuberosity. It is capable of exerting the combination of depression and extension, along with external rotation, and this is a vital contribution since it allows the greater tuberosity to swing beneath the coracoacromial arch during abduction. When this tendon is injured or interfered with as in severe sprain, tear, partial tear or degeneration, circumduction is obstructed because the humerus may jam or rub on the overhanging arch. The external rotation action of the muscle is aided by the rhomboids because of their action of fixing the scapula. When the scapula is flattened against the posterior chest wall, the humerus can more easily be rotated.

THE ANTERIOR PORTION OF THE CUFF is formed by the subscapularis and controls it through a broad, flat muscle belly located on the inner surface of the scapula. The tendon is intimately adherent to the capsule in front and below, and its insertion is into the lesser tuberosity of the humerus. The subscapularis acts as an adductor and internal rotator. It also exerts a downward tension depressing the head of the humerus, aiding the supraspinatous and infraspinatous in holding the humeral head in its proper alignment. This snubbing action allows the other muscles to perform their duties smoothly in their actions on the various movements of the arm. The subscapularis also acts as an "active" ligament helping to hold the humeral head in the glenoid cavity. If the attachment of the subscapularis to the scapula becomes lax or over tense, it may have an effect on the position of the head in the glenoid cavity causing other muscles to react and produce symptoms of shoulder disorders.

The tendons of the rotator muscles are under constant tension on the top, front and back, which in turn favors sprain, tear and wear and tear damage. When a weakness or tear appears, it usually becomes progressively worse because of the multidirectional pull produced by the musculotendinous cuff. Even without arm movement, a constant tension is exerted by the superior portion of the cuff while maintaining the humeral head in proper relationship to the glenoid cavity.

Degenerative changes in the cuff are not uncommon after middle age; most are found in those who do manual work and may cause but slight symptoms. The onset of the situation may be insidious and the cause virtually unknown. The case history will usually indicate some long ago injury ranging from a major sprain to repeated overstrains or other minor events. The supraspinatous portion of the cuff is most frequently affected. It is inserted into the highest part of the tuberosity of the humerus where it is particularly exposed to repeated minor injuries. When the arm is abducted in a medial rotation, the tendon impinges on the acromion and the coracoacromial ligament thereby making it more vulnerable to injury.

CHANGES AND CONDITIONS THAT ARE KNOWN TO OCCUR IN THE CUFF:

1. Degeneration of the tendinous fibers is the earliest pathological change that occurs. As the situation progresses, the entire cuff, joint capsule and biceps tendon may gradually be involved. The tissue becomes edematous and there is diffuse round cell infiltration followed by fibrosis which reduces or prevents all joint movements. This does not happen in all cases and in some it may occur only to a small degree.

The question arises as to what the chiropractic profession can do in these situations and it is the writer's hope that at least some of the answers will be found in these pages.

For the best results it is naturally desirable that the patient should come under care in the early stages. The cause of this type of lesion is, for the most part, occupational strain. There may or may not be a history of trauma. It is the opinion of the writer that the greatest single contributing factor to the onset of this syndrome is that it is caused by the contraction of the muscle bellies by overuse or misuse. This causes tension and strain upon the tendons of the cuff. By palpation, the tension and tenderness can easily be elicited in the muscles. We must take into consideration the vertebral subluxations, most often in the cervical area, and the possibility of referred pain from remote regions or organs. In any event, the supraspinatous, infraspinatous, subscapularis and teres minor must be specifically adjusted or manipulated along with all of the muscles attached to the scapula.

Another very important area to be checked is the head of the humerus, which is often found to be subluxated, placing undue strain upon the musculo-tendinous cuff. Moves correcting these lesions will be shown later in the book.

2. CALCIFIED DEPOSITS are frequently found in the tissues when cuff degeneration occurs. Some are microscopic in size, others large enough to show on x-ray examination, and some may grow to considerable dimensions. According to medical authorities, a medium sized deposit can be seen at operation projecting through the musculo-tendinous cuff into the floor of the subacromial bursa, looking somewhat like a pimple with a yellowish center, surrounded by a ring of hyperemia. It is often extruded like toothpaste from a tube. Deposits may discharge spontaneously into the bursa giving immediate relief, and the calcified material is rapidly absorbed.

The chiropractic doctor will discover this situation through x-ray examination and advise the patient accordingly. Surgery gives the quickest relief from the intense pain and it is hardly advisable to tell the patient to wait until the calcified material discharges and absorbs since this may take a long time or may not happen at all.

Another method used by the medical profession is the injection therapy. This is accomplished by the infiltration of the subacromial area and aspiration of the deposit. This method is fairly satisfactory when the deposit is a fluffy, cloud-like substance, but not all cases respond to it.

3. PARTIAL TEARS of the musculo-tendinous cuff are found most often in the supraspinatous portion and is of considerable clinical importance. However, a tear may occur in any of the tendons that have already begun to degenerate. The case history may indicate that the injury could have been a trivial tear of the deep fibers of the tendon, and this produces few symptoms. A tear of the superficial fibers involves the floor of the bursa, causing it to become inflamed and extremely painful.

4. COMPLETE RUPTURE of the musculo-tendinous cuff is usually due to injury. Occasionally it is a gradual occurrence, sometimes after an injury that was thought to have healed normally. It is the supraspinatous portion of the cuff that is most frequently affected by this tear. However, it may also extend into the infraspinatous and subscapularis portions. The tear in the cuff forms a communication between the joint and the bursa thus exposing the head of the humerus. In time the articular cartilage over this area

becomes eroded and there may be new bone formation at the periphery, giving the appearance of osteoarthritis.

Concealed tears are, without a doubt, the most difficult to detect. The musculo-tendinous cuff is a thick grouping of the tendons, converging into the capsule from different areas of the scapula, inserting into the humerus in order to perform the varying actions of the arm. The construction of this mechanism is such that it allows the deep fibers to be torn while the superficial layers remain intact. The rupture of the deep fibers is called the concealed tear.

Bateman states: "It is a more common lesion than has previously been appreciated, and many shoulders have been explored in the past and closed without the true pathology being recognized." This statement points up the difficulty encountered when arriving at a specific diagnosis in cuff lesions of this type.

5. TEARS OF THE ROTATOR CUFF AND BICIPITAL TEARS are not uncommon in severe accidents and dislocations of the shoulder. The long head of the biceps arises from the scapula just above the glenoid cavity and passes across the upper part of the joint within the capsule and then emerges between the greater and lesser tuberosities and lies in the bicipital groove. It is not directly connected with the capsule as are the tendons of the rotator cuff and it has the added duty of acting as an accessory ligament.

These combined tears most often lie anteriorly over the long head of the biceps. The anterior zone of the capsule covering the head of the humerus is less protected by the coracoacromial arch than the lateral and posterios parts, therefore backward falls put major stress on this area of the capsule and the related tendons. The biceps acts to prevent an upward displacement of the humerus and assumes the function of protection in such falls. When extreme force is applied, the cuff may give way anteriorly, since the infraspinatous exerts a much stronger pull than the supraspinatous. This powerful traction may result in uncovering a large part of the anterior zone of the humeral head and the transverse humeral ligament may become involved as well. This ligament contributes toward the maintenance of the bicipital tendon in its groove. Rotatory stress in particular causes stretching in this area and abduction and external rotation may completely rupture the retaining fibers as the tendon jumps from its groove. Less severe strain weakens this area and allows increased play of the tendon, and a small defect may cause the usual cuff tension, and finally the cuff gives way causing a double lesion of the cuff and bicipital tendon.

The shoulder presents many facets of pain, discomfort and disability. The rotator cuff is, without question, involved directly or indirectly in a great number of shoulder lesions. A traumatized cuff is considered the chief cause of bursitis and tendinitis.

SYMPTOMS OF A RUPTURED MUSCULOTENDINOUS OR ROTATOR CUFF:

Rotator cuff damage is quite common and concealed tears, partial tears and small tears are too often overlooked. The diagnostic signs of a complete rupture are much simpler to ascertain than the three first mentioned injuries and the case history will almost invariably show a person at or close to middle age, one who has had an accident, most often a slip and a fall where he instinctively protected himself by extending his arm.

At times the weight of the body lands on the elbow partially breaking the impact of the fall. The force is transmitted to the shoulder joint and surrounding tissues, or the person may fall so that the shoulder itself takes the full force of the impact. When he regains the standing posture after the accident, he is aware of pain and finds that he cannot lift the arm from his side and that all movements are painful. He is then willing to seek professional help, but some hardy souls wait until the next day.

At this stage he is nearly always unable to dress himself and is in obvious distress, holding the injured arm carefully at the side, supporting it with the other hand. There is generally little or no evidence of external trauma. Palpation over the upper part of the humerus will reveal extreme tenderness. The front and back of the humerus will also be very tender but the pain is not nearly as severe as at the top, in the area of the greater tubercle (Figs. 20-21-22).

In slender patients, an area of depression can be seen in front of the acromion. This would indicate the site of rupture, and many times a clicking sensation can be felt at the top of the shoulder as the humerus rotates under the arch. The clicking is accompanied by a painful catch. When the patient is asked to lift the injured arm, he is able to move it but a short distance when the arm collapses and drops by his side. The effort to abduct the arm is accomplished by bending the head and neck to the opposite side. An effort is made to bring the scapula into play through a jumping action of the shoulder region. When the doctor lifts the arm, an almost normal range of movement can be shown. However, as the humeral head presses under the acromial arch, pain occurs (Figs. 23 and 24).

83

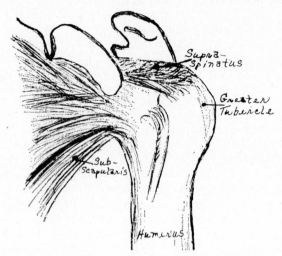

Ant. View of Rotator Cuff and Top of Capsule. Left Shoulder.

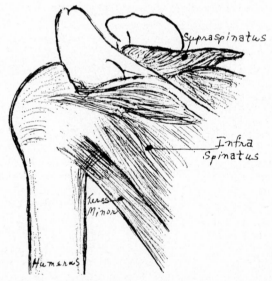

Posterior View of Rotator Cuff and Capsule. Left Shoulder.

Fig. 20

In ten to twelve days there is less pain but more stiffness and the patient may be able to raise the arm about twenty-five degrees, due to the greater help from the accessory abductors. The patient should be examined while sitting since, if he is lying on his back, the doctor could be misled by the apparent power in the cuff, because in that position the scapula is stabilized by the pressure of the body weight which, in turn, would improve deltoid action. In all injuries of this type the doctor should be watchful for a thinning or depression at the fossae of the supra and infraspinatous muscles and also for any signs of deterioration in them because, IN MOST CASES, THIS IS THE CARDINAL SYMPTOM OF A RUPTURED TENDON.

Ordinary x-rays are generally not very helpful in the study of cuff injuries. However, they should be taken and examined carefully in order to locate an abnormality or pathology. Arthrography is relatively new but is of great help in the diagnosis of shoulder lesions. In this method a defect is readily visible, due to diffuse distributions of the dye leaking through an aperture in the cuff and into the subacromial or bicipital areas. The arthrogram also demonstrates an intact capsule with no subacromial leak. Since few chiropractic offices handle this type of x-ray, it would be rather advisable to refer the patient to someone who has the ability and equipment for this type of work in questionable cases. Then there would be no possible doubt as to the diagnosis of a ruptured cuff.

The writer has found from experience that it is advisable in all shoulder complaints and injuries, to take comparative x-rays. It is surprising how many questionable, but apparent defects can be ruled out as causative factors when they also appear in the painless shoulder. Then, too, it is remarkable how many humeral misalignments one will discover in shoulder complaints that are not palpable. More will be discussed on this subject later in the book.

A completely torn tendon must be repaired surgically and it is up to the doctor to do his utmost in making a sound diagnosis so that he can advise correctly in order to produce the optimum results for the patient.

Dr. Bateman, in his book, "THE SHOULDER AND ENVIRONS," states as follows: "The best treatment for a torn tendon anywhere in the body is restoration of its continuity first and then careful re-education of its action complex. These are the principles applied in tears of the rotator cuff also. Most of the confusion and many of the unsatisfactory results in treating these cases are due to inaccurate diagnosis. If the cuff is not torn through its substance completely, recovery will follow good conservative treatment. If there is a definite defect, completely through the cuff, such as may be demonstrated in the arthrogram, operative repair is the method of choice. Once these general principles are clear, discussion of the various factors and situations which modify this general plan is possible."

"Cuff tears occur in middle life or later because the wear and tear degeneration from constant use weakens the tendon. Workmen, particularly in the vulnerable age group, are susceptible to cuff ruptures. A considerable number of tears are encountered after the age of sixty years so that the general condition of the patient, extent and type of tear, occupation, age of the lesion, operative and postoperative facilities are to be considered. Common sense application and interpretation of these factors is all that is necessary. All complete ruptures, that is involving the whole thickness of the tendon, should be repaired when circumstances permit."

The writer believes that Dr. Bateman gives a very concise and common sense summary in the above two paragraphs.

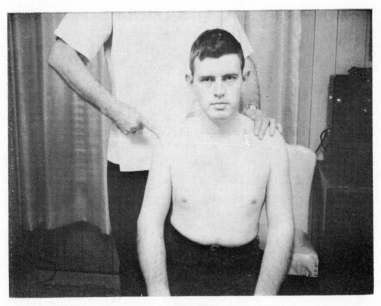

Fig. 21

This picture shows the point of greatest tenderness in ruptures of the rotor cuff.

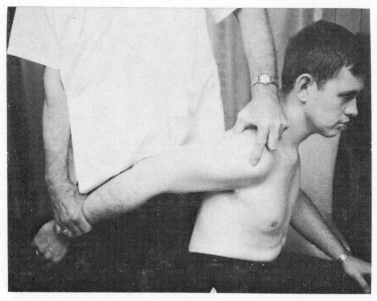

Fig. 22

This shows the method of palpating the humerus in checking for cuff tears. With the arm in the position shown, the doctor's thumb pushes the humeral head farther out from the acromion and the finger is able to palpate the cuff.

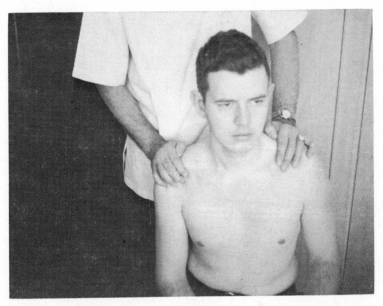

Fig. 23

Testing for a superior subluxation of the humerus in rotor cuff ruptures and long head of the biceps. In this situation the humeral head tends to subluxate to a higher level than normal. X-ray and compare with the un-injured arm.

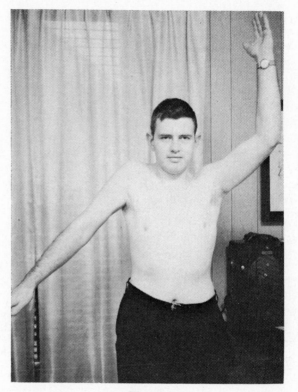

Fig. 24

This shows the typical stance of a person with a ruptured rotor cuff when asked to raise both arms. Note the hunched shoulder. In these situations there is great loss of power.

DEGENERATIVE TENDINITIS

The chief symptom of degenerative tendinitis is pain which the patient will localize by placing his hand and finger tips firmly over the point of the shoulder. Shortly after the onset of the pain, a catching discomfort is felt when lifting the arm. Gradual limitation of movement follows, particularly in rotation. Pain in everyday work increases until it becomes a constant, gnawing ache. As a rule, no significant accident or acute incident, such as overwork, is associated with the cause of this syndrome. The patient will complain of aching at night and difficulty in finding a comfortable position in which to sleep.

Later the pain will appear lower on the arm in the area of the insertion of the deltoid muscle. When the situation progresses to the stage where the pain is so severe that the hair cannot be combed, the back pocket cannot be reached and a night's sleep impossible, then the patient will come to the doctor's office seeking relief. This syndrome most commonly affects the middle aged painter, mason, mechanic, barber, beautician and housewife.

Upon examination, a typical, painful catch is elicited as the arm is lifted and rotated and reaches the point where the humeral head moves under the acromial arch. At this stage the shoulder is not frozen but there is some limitation of movement. The patient may state that he feels something slipping and grinding as the arm is lifted. External and internal rotation are slightly limited and there may be a small amount of atrophy of the supraspinatous, infraspinatous and the deltoid.

Atrophy is never so severe at this stage as when the lesion has progressed to the frozen shoulder stage or when there has been a complete rupture of the cuff (Figs. 23 and 24). Tenderness is present directly over the upper end of the humerus, but the area of maximum tenderness is over the cuff, not over the biceps tendon or the acromion process. The tenderness over the cuff in degenerative tendinitis is quite severe but not as intensely sore as in tendinitis with calcification. There is no complaint of pain along the front of the shoulder or down the medial region of the arm. The patient will usually grasp the shoulder and try to point out the pain. When it has been in evidence for any length of time, the root of the neck and the posterior area of the shoulder also become tender and it may extend to the elbow. In all of these cases the cervical and upper dorsal areas must be examined for subluxations and adjusted, for if the proper treatment is not applied, the situation will continue to worsen until a typical frozen shoulder develops.

INJURIES OF THE BICIPITAL TENDON

In injuries of the bicipital tendon, the long head of the biceps tendon is affected by all movements of the humerus in the glenoid cavity. By its position it contributes much more to shoulder action than only the anchorage of a powerful muscle. There are many avenues of damage to the bicipital apparatus. It is subject to much daily stress and strain, particularly in those individuals who do overhead work. It is the stabilizer of the head of the humerus in front and bears the impact of injuries, especially in backward falls where the arm is extended involuntarily for protection.

Bicipital injuries usually have characteristic symptoms which differ from other shoulder injuries and they are as follows:

1. In taking the case history, the patient will usually recall varying degrees of trauma and these may have been minor in nature or merely overuse. Many persons in the professions who are not accustomed to using their arms, decide to take up a hobby, for example, woodworking. By becoming overly enthusiastic and staying with it for too long a time, muscles that are not accustomed to the activity and not in condition to take the stress and strain, become overworked. The extensive use of a screwdriver or similar tool can produce insult to the bicipital tendon while lifting and pulling heavy objects may also precipitate the discomfort.

2. The patient will complain of pain specifically localized to the shoulder. It will be persistent with all movements of the arm but the forearm and hand are not involved though some pain may radiate from the shoulder for a short distance along the inside of the upper arm. This is, of course, related to the long head of the biceps. Later, weakness and limitation of movement will appear. This is often accompanied by a sharp, painful snapping sensation when the arm is moved. Usually, upon examination, this snap can be felt as well as heard and a persistent general ache will be present. Later, pain and weakness will follow and all rotatory movements will then be carefully avoided. Many times the patient will come to the office in the later stages of his disability and will have his arm close to the side, supporting it with the good hand. The patient learns that the forearm and hand can be used somewhat in this position since it stabilizes the tendon in its groove.

3. Upon examination, the doctor will find the tenderness located at and related to the bicipital mechanism (Fig. 26). The tender area definitely differs from that found in the musculotendinous lesion or calcified tendinitis. In some injuries the tendon may be slack and literally glide from side to side. This can be detected by

placing the finger on the tendon and adducting and externally rotating the arm.

4. Another test for bicipital irregularity may be found by placing the arm on the examining doctor's knee. Then with the hand on the bicipital groove, rotate the arm outward and forward. Instruct the patient to resist this movement. In this way a jumping of the tendon may often be detected (Fig. 27 and 28).

BICIPITAL TENDINITIS AND TENOSYNOVITIS

The bicipital area is not as vulnerable to the syndrome as are the elbow and wrist. Therefore tendinitis and tenosynovitis develop gradually. The long head of the biceps follows a hemmed in course from its origin in the belly of the muscle to the supraglenoid tubercle. Reaction from overuse and strain may occur both in the tendon and its sheath.

The symptoms of bicipital tendinitis and tenosynovitis usually follows a period of activity for which the patient was not conditioned. Playing a game of tennis, strain from unusual forms of lifting or gardening are some of the common culprits.

The patient, when he appears in the doctor's office, will keep the affected arm close to his side with the elbow flexed and he states that he cannot lift any object. Upon palpation, tenderness will be elicited at the top and front of the humerus at an area of the tendon's path across the upper end of the humeral head. Soreness is found along the course of the tendon and into the arm where it can be traced to the bicipital groove. Deep pressure will also show tenderness at the medial border of the deltoid muscle.

In tendinitis or tenosynovitis abnormalities are not likely to be found, however, x-rays may be of value and it is wise to include them in the examination. The films should be taken so that the bicipital groove is clearly outlined. It is also advisable to take a film of the normal shoulder for comparison. These x-rays are taken for the purpose of determining whether or not the groove is too flat, which would allow the tendon to slip, or too deep, which would squeeze and roughen it. The film should also be checked for spur formation (Fig. 25).

CARE OF BICIPITAL TENDINITIS AND TENOSYNOVITIS

This type of syndrome responds very well to chiropractic care. The cervical and upper dorsal regions of the spine need careful checking and adjustments given where the subluxations are found.

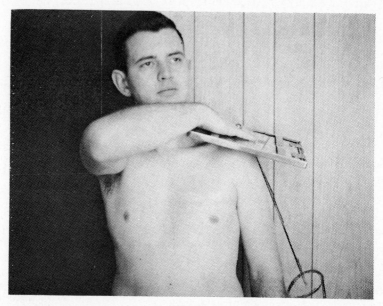

Fig. 25

Here demonstrated is the placement of the casette when making a film to show the bicipital groove. The cone and direction of the central ray are diagrammed in.

All muscles that originate from the scapula and insert into the humerus should be checked for tenderness and contracture. Because of their position and action, the supraspinatous and infraspinatous are usually involved, and the first rib is nearly always subluxated to the superior.

The first rib adjustment is shown in Figs. 62, 63 and 64; the supraspinatous adjustment in Figs. 92, 93 and 94; and the adjustment of the infraspinatous in Figs. 95, 96, 97 and 98. After adjusting, the arm must be immobilized by taping as shown in Figs. 49, 50, 51 and 52, and then placed in a sling because the weight of the arm alone can cause the patient much discomfort. The tape should remain for a period of from three to five days, depending upon its tolerance by the patient's skin. The arm should be carried in a sling for a week to ten days and after the seventh day it should be removed from the sling for short periods of time so that exercises can be instituted, beginning with a gentle one as shown in Figs. 136, 137 and 138. The patient should be encouraged to start active movement after the acute stage is over in order to prevent freezing of the articulation.

If the symptoms continue or increase, the syndrome may be more than a mild tenosynovitis or traumatic tendinitis. It could well be a severe lesion causing the bicipital disturbance, such as a rupture or partial rupture of the tendon. However, the case history, condition and age of the patient should give the doctor sufficient clues regarding the severity of the situation. The majority of cases will respond quickly, but if the doctor finds that it is a complete tendon rupture, surgery will be required to restore its integrity.

RUPTURE OF THE TRANSVERSE HUMERAL LIGAMENT

The transverse humeral ligament is a broad band, passing from the lesser to the greater tubercle of the humerus. It converts the intertubercular groove into a canal. The long head is retained in the groove by it and by a fibrous prolongation from the tendon of the pectoralis major. These are strong fibers blending with the capsule and may rupture or partially rupture when the tendon is placed under great stress. The movements that place the most strain on these fibers are abduction and external rotation. A heavy lift, or a slip while carrying a heavy object, puts a strain on the tendon, and it would slip out of the groove except for the fact that the transverse ligament acts as a checkrein and contains it forcibly in the groove.

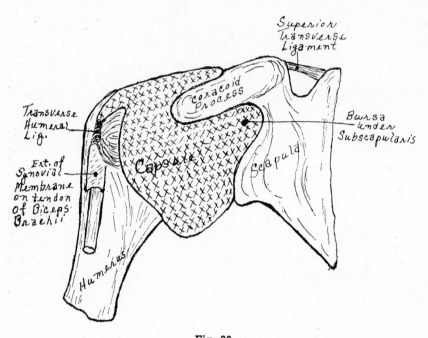

Fig. 26
Capsule of Shoulder Joint (Distended)
Anterior Aspect   (Gray)

96

The injury to the ligament usually occurs when the biceps are flexed and a simultaneous force is exerted as in, for example, Indian wrestling. The writer remembers one case in particular, involving this sport, probably because he was called to the office late at night. Two large, powerful men were wrestling in this manner at a bar for drinks. When they were wrestling for the fourth round of drinks, the injured man said that he felt something snap and the arm gave way. Upon examining the patient, tenderness was found along the route of the tendon but the maximum tenderness was located over the top of the bicipital groove.

In cases such as this, it is best to follow the following procedure: Have the patient sit down. Then the doctor sits in such a manner so that he can place his knee under the patient's arm. The fingers of one hand are placed upon the tendon, his other arm on the patient's forearm and in this manner abduct and internally rotate the arm. A snapping sensation can be felt as the tendon slips back and forth (Fig. 28). However, it will not stay in place without support and if the ligament is completely ruptured, surgical repair will be required (Fig. 26).

The patient referred to in the above paragraph was put through these tests and it was ascertained that he had a torn transverse ligament along with severe injury to the biceps tendon and he was advised to see an orthopedic surgeon.

There may be occasions when a rupture of the fibers of the ligament is part of an anterior tear of the musculotendinous cuff. All cases are not as severe as the one mentioned in the previous paragraph. There are many instances of strain on the intertubercular fibers which, however, need the proper case management to prevent the patient from suffering later damage. The shoulder should be taped as shown in Figs. 49, 50, 51 and 52, and the arm placed in a sling for approximately two weeks; the taping allowed to remain for three to five days and the patient instructed to avoid flexion and external rotation. This type of injury is generally found in younger persons. Active movement should be encouraged as soon as the acute pain subsides, as described in the chapter on exercises.

RUPTURES OF THE BICEPS TENDON, ROTOR CUFF AND NERVE DAMAGE

This is a very serious injury and involves rupture of the biceps tendon, extensive damage to the musculotendinous cuff and a varying degree of nerve damage which can cause partial brachial paralysis. It may also involve a subluxation or dislocation of the head of the humerus.

This injury usually occurs in older persons. The patient slips and falls backward. The arm is outstretched and involuntarily placed behind for protection. In this manner the head of the humerus is forced forward and upward. The stress is taken on the long head of the biceps, the capsule and the antero-medial ligaments and muscles. There will be extensive ecchymosis over the anterior and medial portion of the shoulder and chest area, indicating extensive soft tissue damage and injury to the neurovascular bundle.

Chiropractically, the subluxations and dislocations of the shoulder must be corrected and the nerve injuries alleviated. The tendon and cuff damage may remain disabling and surgery on the torn tendon may be properly advised, depending on the age and condition of the patient.

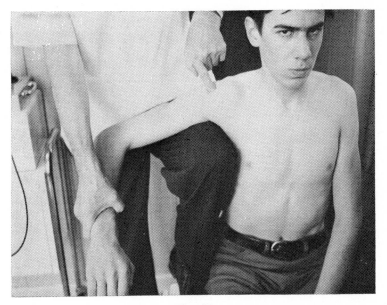

Fig. 27

This photograph shows the palpation of the transverse humeral ligament to determine the presence of strain, partial tear or complete rupture of the ligament and tendon of the long head of the biceps. The forearm is moved up and down on the doctor's knee to ascertain the amount of tenderness and the degree of movement of the bicipital tendon.

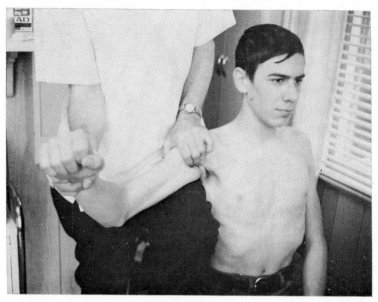

Fig. 28

One of the doctor's hands is placed over the area of the bicipital groove as shown while the patient's arm is laid across the doctor's knee. He then grasps the patient's wrist with the other hand. Then the doctor works his fingers under the short head of the biceps and coracobrachialis to compress the bicipital tendon, and pushes the patient's forearm down at the same time instructing the patient to resist the downward pressure. If a jumping sensation is detected over the tendon, it would indicate a partial tear of the transverse humeral ligament. If, on the other hand, a gliding sensation is felt going out of the bicipital groove, it would indicate a torn transverse ligament.

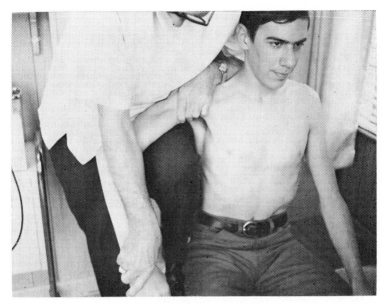

Fig. 29

THE ADJUSTMENT OF THE BICIPITAL TENDON

If the ligament is still strong enough to hold the tendon at least partially in the groove, it is subluxated and can be adjusted. However, supportive measures, as shown in Figs. 49, 50, 51 and 52, must be used along with a sling.

First, place the patient, and the doctor should place his hands, as shown in the PRECEDING photograph. The above picture shows the position of the doctor and patient's arm when the adjustive force is completed. Instruct the patient NOT to resist since the move is not painful.

Then the doctor places a firm contact over the muscles, as described, and brings the patient's forearm straight forward and down very quickly. This adjustment will be found to be very beneficial in the painful sprains, strains and contractures and brings almost immediate relief.

In case of a completely torn ligament, this method can be used to replace it into the bicipital groove. However, even with the best supportive measures, it will not stay and surgery should be advised.

101

FIBROSITIS

Whenever there are severe neck and shoulder pains, a large percentage of musculotendinous disorders are diagnosed as fibrositis. In a majority of these cases the symptoms are of a gradual onset, characterized by a gnawing, aching type of pain. The patient will indicate the general area by placing the palm of the hand between the neck and shoulder.

No severe trauma will be indicated in the case history. The patient will usually complain of a gradual buildup of pressure or tension in the neck and scapular area. Palpation will elicit pain, tension and stringiness in the affected muscles, and some crepitus may also be detected. In acute cases, whole segments of the muscles are prominent in spasm which will persist even in the relaxed posture.

The muscles most commonly affected are the trapezius, levator scapulae, the scalene group, particularly the anticus and medius, the upper part of the sacro-spinalis or erector spinea, the rhomboids and the supra and infraspinatous. The adjustment and specific manipulations of these muscles will be discussed later in the book under the heading "Specific Muscular Manipulation."

From this area, pain radiates up the back of the neck and out over the shoulder, and occasionally reaching the upper part of the arm. No acute distress is associated with either shoulder or neck action, however, a vague soreness is experienced with both neck and shoulder movements.

The chief cause of fibrositis is poor posture, occupational strain and minor trauma causing tension and spasm in the group of aforementioned muscles. Although fibrositis is a term used to describe a disturbance in soft tissue producing symptoms of pain, stiffness and, to a degree, a limitation of movements, any part under stress may involve the muscle fascia, tendons, ligaments or fibrous supporting tissue. The chiropractor need not be reminded of their importance to the spinal subluxation in the treatment of this lesion.

The patients who seek relief from fibrositis are in the main women, between thirty and fifty years of age. Their complaint is of pain between the shoulders and out over the shoulder area. They may be in the menopause, usually undernourished, frail, and may complain of being nervous or worried. Many times they may have a chronic illness which aggravates the situation. Their discomfort is worse in the morning or following any period of inactiviy. There

102

apparently is some relief when the muscles are used and warmed. It is difficult to pinpoint any one cause; chronic strain, minute trauma, focal infection, heredity, postural habits and occupational strain are all contributing factors.

Dr. Bateman states in his book as follows: "Thickening in the muscles is encountered related to the points of maximum tenderness. Sometimes this is a fairly definitely demarcated nodule but more often it is a diffuse fullness without clear-cut margins and may not seem to be the same area of muscle palpated each time. When a definite nodule is present and is excised, it appears composed of fibrofatty or fibrous tissue replacing muscle. Sometimes only a little infiltrating fibrosis with atrophy of muscle fibers is present.

"Many of these dense areas in muscles have been explored without much pathology being found. This is explained on the basis of spasm in the muscle which is the prominent finding in the early stage before structural change has occurred. It seems logical to accept the 'fibrositic lesion' as the guise of musculofascial reaction to many irritants and to anticipate differences in the lesion corresponding to the phases and degrees of the process. When a definite nodule is found, it is a fibrofatty herniation through the superficial fascia."

Most of these cases respond remarkably well under chiropractic care. The muscles in the involved area should be manipulated, lightly in the beginning and gradually increasing in intensity. However, when a palpable trigger point is found, it is best to avoid contact on it until the patient shows some improvement because many of these persons have a low pain threshold. The patient should be prepared by the doctor to accept the muscle soreness which will occur after the first few adjustments and be told to use hot baths or hot packs if it is more than minor.

The patient should be advised on proper dietary habits and in the frail person, a diet to produce a weight gain would be very beneficial. Since drafts or chilling from an inadequate amount of clothing will nearly always have an adverse effect on persons in this situation, they should be instructed to keep themselves warm at all times. Their postural faults must be corrected, including sleeping habits. They should have a firm mattress and avoid sleeping face down with the head turned to the side. Finally, the doctor should provide a light exercise program geared to the individual. Isometric exercises have been found to be very beneficial to these patients.

103

THE FROZEN SHOULDER

The painful, contracted or frozen shoulder is one of the most difficult of all shoulder cases with which to cope, though its diagnosis is simple. Frozen shoulder is a blanket term covering many ills and the difficult part for the doctor is to identify the underlying cause since we seldom see the condition in its primary stage. Because the onset is almost always gradual, the patient hopes that it will "go away" and so does not seek help until the condition is in its terminal stage of near or complete uselessness of the affected arm.

The conditions contributing to a frozen shoulder are tindinitis of the rotator cuff, bicipital lesions, acromioclavicular arthritis and cuff tears. There is no single etiological factor but rather a combination of pathologies and it is important to find the true, underlying cause. Most commonly, this condition arises from a gradual degeneration in the rotator cuff or bicipital mechanism.

Typically, the patient is forty-five years of age or older and comes to the office complaining of severe pain localized in the shoulder area. He will state that it has been present for some time and that it has become most acute at night. Arm movements aggravate the pain and relief is obtained by not using it. Because of the disuse, stiffening progressively becomes worse and eventually the normal free swinging of the arm and shoulder is entirely lost. The accessory muscles are then brought into use in order to partly overcome the deficient shoulder movement and the pain then becomes prominent also in the posterior region of the neck and shoulder due to the increased strain on this group of muscles.

Examination will show that the head of the humerus is adhesed to the glenoid cavity and for that reason this lesion is also referred to as adhesive capsulitis. The movement of the humerus in the glenoid cavity is lost and the only movement that can be accomplished is through the shifting of the whole shoulder girdle upon the chest wall. Adduction and rotation are at times almost non-existent and there is atrophy of all of the muscles around the shoulder. The degree of atrophy is directly proportional to the length of time that the person has had the condition. There is tenderness upon palpation at the superior, anterior and lateral aspects of the humerus and it is difficult to pinpoint the area of maximum tenderness since the whole of the affected shoulder is extremely sore.

Unfortunately, x-ray films of a frozen shoulder too often give but little information concerning the changes that have taken place. However, they should nonetheless be taken in order to ascertain whether or not there is arthritis, osteoporosis or other pathological condition in the glenoid and humeral head. Again it is stressed that comparative films be made of both shoulders for the reasons previously stated. In the majority of cases, the head of the humerus will be found subluxated superiorly on the affected side. It is not advisable to attempt correction of this subluxation until at least a partial release of the muscle spasms has been accomplished. Severe, shotgun manipulation can do more harm than good.

PATHOLOGY OF THE FROZEN SHOULDER

Dr. Bateman, in his book, gives a very interesting and informative description of findings during operative procedures and he is quoted as follows:

"In a relatively early and acute case at operation, the synovium is stuck to articular cartilage and needs to be pulled from the surface, giving away in the same fashion adhesive tape does from any smooth surface. Normal intra-articular space is almost completely obliterated and the joint cavity is filled with the juicy, redundant, injected lining. The normal lax, pleat-like folding at the inferior aspect is lost as the synovial surfaces become glued together. The capsule becomes thickened and contracted also limiting movement. The muscle layers, tense and spastic from pain stimulation, remain contracted and later atrophy. As the joint structures contract, layer by layer, the freezing process becomes complete. In later stages, the adhesions become thick and fixed, tying capsule to bone. The joint cavity is dry and small and the head of the humerus is drawn up close to the glenoid.

"These changes are not indolent, passive degeneration and are not the result of lack of movement only. The appearance of degenerative tendinitis differs profoundly from this lesion, and those joints, the seat of paralytic disorder, never appear like this although movement may have been absent for a long time. There is some independent active change setting off the profound synovial condition; probably capsule and muscle response are secondary to the lining irritation. Some antecedent episode can normally be unearthed but a percentage may be regarded as an idiopathic adhesive capsulitis. This is the term which should be reserved for the condition because it most accurately depicts the pathological picture. Periarthritis is much too general and would include a multitude of lesions.

"In the late stages, more profound changes are found in the capsular and extra-capsular structures. The rotor cuff is thick and inelastic; the biceps tendon frequently glued to its groove, and the normal synovial lining sleeve protection is completely obliterated. The subacromial bursa is thin, dry and brittle. Tough adhesions traverse the subacromial space at the margins of the bursa. These are firmly implanted in the cuff, usually at the musculotendinous junction. These adhesions are so strong and firmly attached that they may pull pieces out of the cuff on rugged manipulation, just as one pulls up soil on the roots of a plant. Accessory ligaments become thickened, gluing joint structures together. The coracohumeral ligament appears as a tight check rein, tautly stretched from the coracoid, holding the humerus in internal rotation."

Dr. Bateman, in describing his procedure and findings in surgery on the frozen shoulder, gives a clear picture of the pathological and structural changes within and around the shoulder joint and it would be well to keep these in mind when treating this type of lesion.

Unscientific, forceful, shotgun manipulation should never be used when adjusting the shoulder. This method of treatment may cause tears in the rotator cuff and other important structures may be badly damaged. Some surgeons have used rugged manipulation while the patient was under anaesthesia but, reportedly, this is no longer done with much frequency. Dr. Bateman says: "Depending upon the enthusiasm of the operator, various results have been reported. Undoubtedly some are helped, but it is felt that these are the ones that would do well under the conscientious conservative regime anyway. In the difficult and quite small group, the author feels blind manipulation does harm and it is preferable to resect the binding adhesions surgically under direct vision."

Note that Dr. Bateman says that a SMALL group need surgery. He also says in his book that good physiotherapy is the basis of treatment and advocated it along with an exercise program for the relief of the frozen shoulder.

Every chiropractic doctor has been confronted with this baffling type of case, and they are never simple or easy to correct. However, it is the writer's opinion that through chiropractic treatment plus common sense manipulation of the accessory muscles, a regime of corrective exercises and good case management, a high percentage of cures and much relief can be obtained for even the most severe of these conditions.

There is no question but that prevention is the best cure for these lesions. Therefore, every painful shoulder problem that presents itself to our offices should be taken seriously and especially so if the patient is over fifty years of age. Older persons are most susceptible and even a mild disturbance, such as a seemingly light blow or bruise to the supraspinatous, tendinitis or bicipital trauma can possibly end in a frozen shoulder.

Though the writer has cared for a large number of frozen shoulders which presented varied case histories, one in particular made a great impression and gave him much added confidence in treating these situations thereafter.

More than twenty years ago the writer was called to the home of a very prominent and wealthy businessman for a consultation. Upon arriving, he was informed that both shoulders were giving the patient much difficulty and upon examination it was found that both were in a severely frozen state. When in the erect position, the patient was unable to comb his hair with either hand and his fingers could be brought up only as far as the earlobes. He was able to go to his office and do desk work by having his chair raised.

The patient did not know of any reason for the onset, stating that it had come on gradually and had simply become progressively worse. He was a very active person of sixty-five. He said that the discomfort had begun in October and by December it was so painful that he had gone to a famous midwestern clinic seeking help. After a complete examination, he was told that there was nothing organically wrong and that he should go home, take it easy and apply heat by means of a "baker" which he had constructed according to directions, by a local appliance shop. The baker consisted of a half round piece of metal long enough to cover his body from the waist to the neck, and having three electric lights on each side. He was told to bake himself twice a day for a half hour each time. This he had been doing faithfully for two months without results and it was now the middle of February.

At this point he was anxious to try chiropractic since he wanted to be well by June first for a reason that was most important to him, namely, lawn bowling. This was a sport that he had introduced to our city and he had been champion for five years. It was his great desire to capture the title once more. The writer took the case with the understanding that, in his opinion, the patient would be able to bowl but with no guarantee that he would retain the championship! He was made to understand that a goodly number

107

of adjustments would be required, that he would be adjusted three times a week and that a regular exercise regime would have to be faithfully followed.

His first exercises were those shown in Figs. 134 and 135. After a week, he was able to start the stretches. In his case, an exercise bar was used, such as can be purchased from an orthopedic supply company, or the stretches can be done as shown in Figs. 140 and 141. His exercise bar was placed in a doorway and he had a sturdy bench constructed to stand on so that he could reach it. He was instructed to grasp it with both hands, then slowly and gradually let some of his body weight down, thus stretching the arms, until his tolerance was reached. He was told to do six consecutive stretches of about ten seconds each twice daily and to increase both the number and length of the stretches as tolerance permitted.

By the third week he had improved to the point where he was able to tolerate twelve to fifteen stretches of twenty seconds each, and no longer needed the bench to stand on. At this point two more exercises were added, the first being a lifting motion. He was told to grasp the under edge of a heavy table and pull upwards, this for the purpose of stretching the muscles from the opposite direction. The second consisted of a swinging motion as shown in Figs. 136 and 137 up to his tolerance, beginning with thirty seconds and gradually increasing the time to several minutes. NOTE: Do not use the exercise described in Fig. 137 after an anterior dislocation.

With the regular adjustments and his complete cooperation in following the prescribed exercises, he was ready to bowl long before his June deadline. He not only again won the championship but also won the free and normal use and movement of his shoulders without any pain or discomfort. This patient never had a recurrence of the condition and he lived to be eighty-five. However, from the time of his recovery, he never failed to stretch his arms and shoulders twice a day on the bar that became a permanent part of his doorway.

In this case, subluxations were found in the cervical and dorsal areas of the spine. No doubt some were primary and some secondary because of the effort encountered when substituting the movement of the shoulder girdle to the accessory muscles in order to compensate for the lack of normal muscle control. The first ribs were superior on both sides, the right one most prominently so, and these were adjusted as shown in Figs. 62 and 63. When only one shoulder is affected, the superior rib will be on that side.

The muscles most severely affected in this patient were the supraspinatous, the levator scapulae, the rhomboids and those portions of the trapezius that are inserted into the scapula. They were all extremely tense and tender and were specifically manipulated as shown in the chapter on muscle adjusting. Along with these, the muscles related to the quadrilateral space were found to be extremely tender and were manipulated as shown in Figs. 75 to 79 inclusive.

Chapter VII
CORRECTIVE METHODS AND CASE MANAGEMENT PROCEDURES

THE ACROMIOCLAVICULAR LESION

There is very little movement in this articulation until the arm has reached an angle of approximately eighty-five degrees. The movements are of two kinds, one a gliding motion of the articular end of the clavicle on the acromion and second, the rotation of the acromial end of the scapula upon the clavicle.

The usual disorders of this joint are sprain, subluxation, dislocation and arthritis. Sprain and subluxations occur rather frequently in industry and athletics, particularly in football where there is a great deal of physical contact.

THE SPRAINED ACROMIOCLAVICULAR JOINT

The sprained acromioclavicular joint is simple to care for. Since there is usually little or no apparent separation, a good supportive taping will generally be sufficient (Fig. 33).

THE ACROMIOCLAVICULAR SEPARATION

This is a common injury and occurs more frequently than the complete dislocation. The subluxation is easily detected by comparison with the uninjured side and the lateral end of the clavicle will appear slightly higher and will be extremely tender upon palpation. With a downward pressure, a slight movement will be detected. This indicates a mild or partial tear of the ligaments. The clavicle should be adjusted since it not only tends to subluxate superiorly but also forward (Fig. 31). The adjustment should be followed by a strong taping over the clavicle and shoulder girdle first, then over the shoulder with the anchorage under the arm as shown in Fig. 35.

It should always be noted whether or not any deformity is present on the uninjured side since many persons have enlarged lateral clavicular ends which could be mistakenly diagnosed as a subluxation. The writer has cared for a great number of these cases and all have terminated in a satisfactory manner through the use of the corrective adjustment, adequate supportive measures and proper case management.

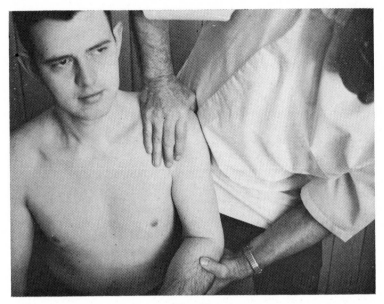

Fig. 30

This photograph shows the method of testing for the presence of an acromio-clavicular separation and the degree to which it is present. The doctor places one hand over the acromio-clavicular joint and holds firm pressure. He places the other under the elbow and pushes up. The more "give" that is felt in the joint, the greater the separation.

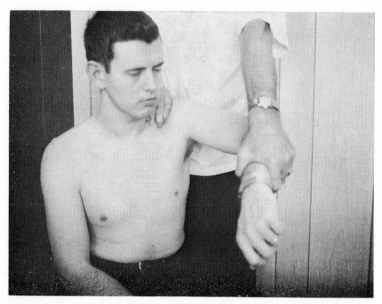

Fig. 31

This picture shows the adjustment used in the acromio-clavicular separation. The doctor places the fingers of one hand over the clavicle and with a
firm pressure moves it downward and inward while simultaneously moving
the arm forward and downward. At the beginning of this move, the elbow
is bent with the hand pointing nearly straight up. When the move is completed, the hand and forearm should be parallel with the floor as shown.
Do NOT move the arm lower than parallel with the floor because the clavicle
could then be moved forward to cause a re-separation.

112

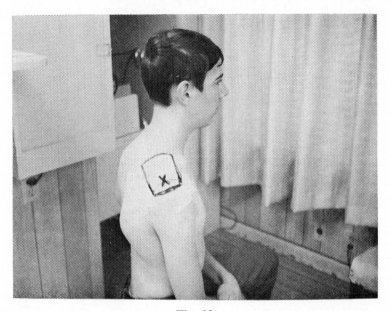

Fig. 32

The above picture shows the first step in the taping for the acromio-clavicular separation. A piece of foam rubber is placed over the articulation, cut to about 3 by 4 inches. It is held in place with a criss-cross taping.

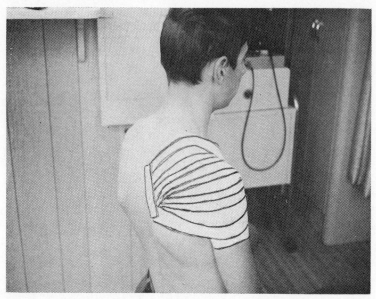

Fig. 33

This photograph shows the completed taping without the sling. The tape is started at the front and the line of tape tension is from front to back. The first piece of tape is placed over the top of the shoulder and successive pieces are placed lower, each with an overlap, until the shoulder and upper arm are supported as shown. Inch and a half width tape is used.

114

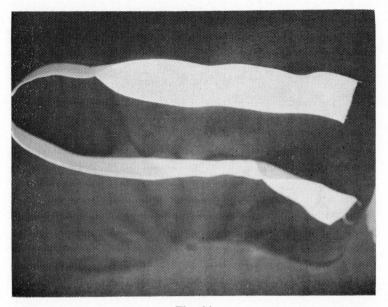

Fig. 34

This picture shows the tape sling. About a yard of inch and a half tape is necessary, depending upon the size of the person. On one end leave about 8 inches unfolded and on the other about 4 inches should be left open and the area between folded in half, sticky sides together. This can be accomplished easily by lightly sticking the tape to the adjusting table—first put the 8 inch area down, then put the 4 inch area down about two feet away, thus forming a loop. Then with the thumb and forefinger squeeze the tape between the fastened down areas together.

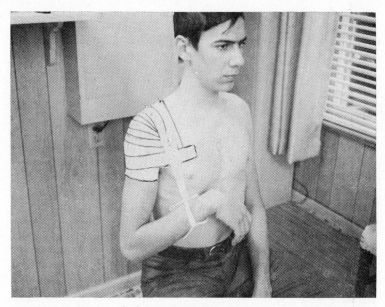

Fig. 35

This picture shows the sling in place. The usual neck sling will not be as effective in this type of condition as the one shown because this method utilizes the weight of the arm to aid in stabilizing the injured articulation and help prevent upward movement of the clavicle. To place the sling start with the 8 inch open end of the tape, place it directly behind the articulation, bring the tape forward and directly OVER the joint. Bring it down and between the body and arm, then around the arm and up so that the arm is in the position shown and the 4 inch area of adhesive is anchored firmly to the folded area of the sling. A foam rubber pad is then placed between the arm and sling, as shown, to prevent the weight of the arm from irritating the tissues. Some team physicians place the sling close to or under the elbow. However, it is the writer's opinion from experience that the placement shown is more effective.

THE ACROMIOCLAVICULAR DISLOCATION

The integrity of the acromioclavicular articulation depends upon the conoid and trapezoid ligaments (Fig. 2). The joint cannot become completely dislocated unless both ligaments are ruptured. Such an injury can be caused by a fall or severe blow on the point of the shoulder. The clinical picture is characterized by the following symptoms: the weight of the arm pulls the acromion downward, the end of the clavicle is prominent and elevated, there is a visible and palpable dropoff between the two and the clavicle can be pressed downward, springing up again when the pressure is released. All of this can easily be seen when compared with the uninjured side.

The complete dislocation is best cared for surgically and since there is a complete tearing of the ligaments, integrity must be restored. The screw fixation method is usually used in which a screw fixes the clavicle to the coracoid process. This method controls the dislocation and corrects the deformity. There is some question regarding the advisability of leaving the screw in place after the fixation period since activity places a strain on it which may cause a loosening. Most authorities recommend that it be removed in from six to eight weeks.

ACROMIOCLAVICULAR ARTHRITIS

The common cause of arthritis in this articulation is not usually primary but rather the result of post traumatic degeneration. This region is quite vulnerable to injury and occupational stress. Since disturbances of this joint produces a localized pain, it may be overlooked or confused with the more common rotor cuff or bicipital lesions.

The overhanging coracoacromial arch is exposed to injury from above and below. This area of the shoulder takes a great deal of abuse when carrying or holding heavy objects and is also subjected to blows and general stresses. These may be damaging because the articulation is not much protected by muscles as are most other parts of the body.

Injury and degeneration are common causes of acromioclavicular arthritis. The condition usually begins with pain in the general shoulder area and the patient will experience difficulty in sleeping and, as a rule, will sleep on the affected side. Activities below shoulder level do not cause too much discomfort, however, intense pain is noted after the arm is raised to a right angle. Movement in this

117

joint does not begin until the scapula starts to rotate with the humerus and the clavicle remains anchored. Therefore, maximum pain and the greatest disability is found in occupations where it is necessary to work with the arms overhead, or at or near a right angle with the body, and this factor distinguishes it from other shoulder disorders. The position in which pain is felt contrasts sharply with cuff lesions such as degenerative tendinitis, where the pain occurs at a lower arm level.

Examination of the superior area of the shoulder will often show irregularity. Upon palpation, tenderness will be located over the joint line and in some cases crepitus may be felt as the arm is abducted above a right angle. In the more advanced cases, a jumping sensation may be felt due to the slipping of the lateral end of the clavicle. Some articulations may appear to be subluxated or dislocated when in reality there is only an enlargement of the end of the clavicle. This may appear without articular damage. A simple test may be made by placing the fingers of one hand on the acromio-clavicular joint and the palm of the other one underneath the elbow. Then, holding a fairly firm pressure on the clavicle, push up on the elbow. This will test the stability of the articulation and also produce pain if it is an acute condition (Fig. 30).

When the contour seems abnormal, and one shoulder is painful, the suspected articulation should be x-rayed as well as the painless shoulder so that an accurate comparison can be made. (It is not uncommon to have both ends of the clavicle slightly enlarged or unusually prominent without producing symptoms.)

When the point of tenderness and area of pain have been located and the joint changes determined by x-ray, the doctor will have little difficulty in differentiating between acromioclavicular arthritis, cuff lesions and bicipital disturbances. X-rays are important in ascertaining the extent to which the articulation is damaged. Most of those types of conditions are the direct cause of trauma or post traumatic degeneration. It is essential, of course, that fracture be completely eliminated before proceding with any treatment.

X-rays should be taken with the patient in the sitting or standing posture so that the weight of the arm pulls on the articulation since a film taken lying down will not show the true degree of separation. Again, films should be taken of both shoulders for comparison. According to Dr. Bateman, a dislocation can best be demonstrated by having the patient standing and facing the tube, with a weight in each hand, the central ray being directed to the sternal notch. The writer believes that this would also be a good method for determining the degree of subluxation in the articulation.

In the rare, extreme cases, it may be necessary to consider the surgical excision of the outer end of the clavicle.

THE STERNOCLAVICULAR JOINT

The relatively small movement of this articulation is nonetheless extremely essential for full shoulder girdle movements, keeping in mind that the medial portion of the clavicle is more securely anchored than is the lateral aspect. Injuries to the sternoclavicular joint are similar to those of the acromioclavicular, namely sprain, subluxation, injury to the intra-articular disc, dislocation and arthritis.

The case history will usually indicate a blow or fall in which the force of impact came from behind and in a lateral direction. Severe falls on the lateral and posterior area of the shoulder usually are the main causes for this type of injury.

THE SPRAINED STERNOCLAVICULAR JOINT

The simple sprain is easily cared for since there is usually no separation, and tenderness will be found over and around the articulation. A proper supportive taping as shown in Fig. 38 is usually sufficient.

THE STERNOCLAVICULAR SUBLUXATION

This is a common injury particularly in football, industry and agriculture, or whenever a person falls and strikes the lateral posterior aspect of the shoulder. The writer has cared for a large number of these cases where the patients were injured as a result of farming accidents—falling from tractors and other implements, thus injuring their shoulders. This type of fall is usually so fast, hard and unexpected that the person does not have time to stretch his arm out to protect himself against the impact. However, the subluxation is easily adjusted as shown in Fig. 36.

After correction, supportive measures must be applied. This is done by taping a pad of rubber or splint (Fig. 37) over the injury. The writer often uses a splint made by cementing foam rubber to a tongue depressor and taping it in place (Figs. 38 and 39). For added stability, a pad of cotton or lamb's wool may be placed in the armpit. The arm should then be placed in a sling, remaining there

119

for a week to ten days. The tape should remain in place for as long as the patient's skin can tolerate it. If the skin becomes irritated, two ace bandages taped together end to end may be used for support as shown in Fig. 40 and 41. If these injuries are taken lightly and are not given the proper case management, the joint can become the site of post-traumatic arthritis.

THE STERNOCLAVICULAR - INTRA-ARTICULAR DISC INJURY

The disc may be injured to such an extent that it can be separated internally from its attachment at the sternum. It may cause internal degrees of derangement or tears similar to the semilunar tears in the knee. This damage can occur in injuries that are less severe than those causing dislocation. The symptoms are pain, a catching sensation on flexion or circumduction of the arm, accompanied by a clicking sensation. If the condition persists, surgery may be necessary to remove the torn pieces of cartilage and for capsule repair.

STERNOCLAVICULAR DISLOCATION

Sternoclavicular dislocations are not common injuries. In these situations the medial end of the clavicle is forced in front of the sternum, being pushed upward and outward. These cases always present a history of severe injury, usually an extremely hard fall. It is rare when the medial aspect of the clavicle is forced beneath the sternum. In a few instances the dislocation can be reduced by the same procedure as that used in the correction of the subluxated clavicle. However, the writer believes that the wisest course is to send them to an orthopedic practitioner because in nearly all cases the pain is excruciating and ligamentous and tissue damage severe.

STERNOCLAVICULAR ARTHRITIS

Sternoclavicular arthritis may follow an injury of the above discussed types. The symptoms of post traumatic arthritis are pain, tenderness and mild swelling. The articulation should be x-rayed in order to ascertain the extent of degeneration and the patient advised accordingly. If the degeneration is extensive and the pain unbearably severe, the medial end of the clavicle may have to be surgically excised, or possibly an excision of the exostosis can be done along with smoothing of the joint margins.

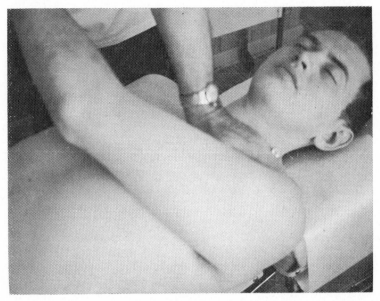

Fig. 36

The above picture shows the adjustment of the subluxated clavicle. The doctor stands on the opposite side of injury, placing the hand over the subluxation. With his other hand he slowly pulls the patient's arm toward himself, simultaneously giving a slight thrust upon the clavicle. Then place the patient's arm across his abdomen and caution him not to move it until the taping is completed (Figs. 38 and 39).

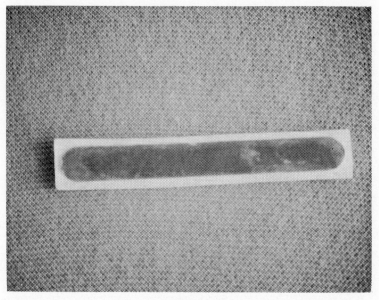

Fig. 37

Pictured above is a splint used in a sterno-clavicular lesion. It is made by cementing a tongue depressor to foam rubber. It should be placed over the injury so that its center is directly on the separation.

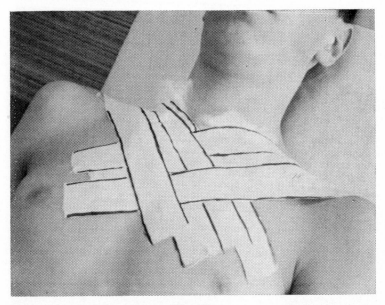

Fig. 38

These photographs show the taping of the sterno-clavicular lesion. First, prepare the splint as shown in Fig. 37 and, with the foam side down, tape it in place over the injury just enough to hold it down. Next, generously place cotton padding in a V shape on either side of, and very close to the neck, also padding the presternal notch. Then tear eight tape strips long enough (depending on the size of the patient) so they will extend on the front chest wall as shown and down the back to about two or three inches below the superior scapular border.

With the patient's arm across his abdomen, begin the taping. Start on the back of the injured side, bringing the tape over and to the front as close as possible to the neck, being sure that the cotton padding protects the skin and muscles. Place the second strip on the uninjured side, the third one again on the injured side and keep alternating in this criss-cross pattern until each side has four strips applied.

As each piece of tape is brought over from the back and across the front, the doctor should push the injured clavicle downward with a firm pressure. The pull of all pieces of tape, except the two lower horizontal anchor strips shown in the following picture, is FROM the back TO the front. In cases of a simple sprain, the above portion of the taping is usually sufficient and the doctor need not complete the steps described next.

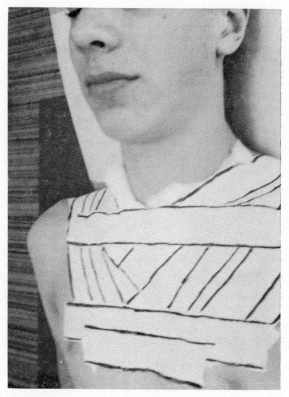

Fig. 39

This shows the completed taping which is done in the same manner as described above, namely to alternate the application of the strips to continue the criss-cross, and keeping the direction of pull from back to front. In this step the "base" of support is widened because five or six strips are used on each side. The lower two horizontal strips are for the purpose of anchorage while the upper one is pressed firmly in place over the site of injury.

The doctor may use even more criss-cross strips if he deems it necessary. The same anchorage shown on the front should be applied to the posterior tape endings. Then the arm is placed in a regular neck sling with a piece of cotton padding in the armpit for added comfort.

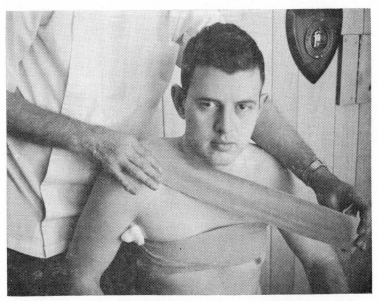

USE OF THE ACE BANDAGE IN CASE MANAGEMENT
Fig. 40

For the wrap here described it is necessary to tape two ace bandages together end to end. This method is used in the latter stages of case management of both the acromio-clavicular and sterno-clavicular lesions. Presuming that the injury is on the right side, start the wrap on the back on the left side of the spine and roll it toward the right, going straight around the body twice and then bringing the wrap up and over the shoulder as shown. At this time, place a three or four-inch square of foam rubber over the site of injury and place a cotton cushion in the armpit.

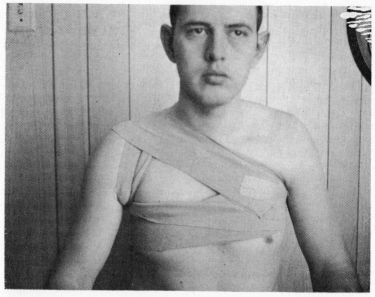

Fig. 41

Next, carry the wrap under the uninjured (left) arm, around the back toward the right side, under the right arm and toward the front, then up and around the shoulder joint. Encircle the shoulder joint a second time. Then bring the wrap down the back of the shoulder to the right armpit, again bringing it to the front and taking it across the front of the chest, around the back diagonally to the right shoulder and over it, then diagonally across the chest and toward the left side. Continue in this manner to the end of the wrap and fasten with tape.

If the doctor wishes to provide added support, three or four strips of tape can be applied over the front, diagonal area of the wrap, starting the tape strips on the upper posterior area of the injured side.

126

Chapter VIII

SHOULDER DISLOCATIONS

There is much speculation concerning the reasons why some dislocations heal and cause no further difficulty while others will give repeated trouble.

Some authorities maintain that the nature of the lesions is different. In the nonrecurring dislocations the head of the humerus passes through a tear in the joint capsule, and this heals readily. In the recurring type, the glenoid ligament is detached and cannot readhere because of the poor blood supply. This view is disputed by other authorities who believe that in the initial lesion, all cases have a detachment of the glenoid ligament. Basically, the repeated dislocations recur because the arm has not been well enough immobilized after reduction of the first traumatic incident or that the succeeding violent accidents just happen to the same previously injured shoulder.

The doctor will encounter several kinds of dislocations:

1. The acute dislocation which may be—
   A. The anterior dislocation
   B. The posterior dislocation
   C. The subglenoid dislocation
2. The recurrent dislocation, either anterior, posterior or subglenoid.
3. The unreduced or chronic dislocation, either anterior, posterior or subglenoid.
4. The compound dislocation where the bone tears through the soft tissues producing an open wound.

The dislocation may be acute, chronic, recurrent, simple or compound and the diagnosis is established on the basis of the case history. A dislocated shoulder may look like a deformity, there being a depression where bone should normally be, or a tumor-like protrusion where it normally should not be. Compare visually and by palpation with the normal side. Note the loss of function, the degree and extent of disability in joint movement and the method of movement; the amount of spasm in the surrounding muscles, the extent of swelling, tenderness and pain.

A definite point or points of extreme pain may suggest fracture, therefore x-ray films are an absolute necessity and no attempt should be made at reduction until the possibility of fracture is definitely eliminated. A lateral x-ray is informationally the most productive. Additional complications to be reckoned with are traumatized arteries, veins and nerves. If circulatory and sensory nerve damage is present there will be coldness and blanching of the skin, or cyanosis, and when the damage is to the motor nerves, paralysis will result.

Prompt reduction of the acute dislocation is most desirable in order to lessen the irritation and resultant inflammation. Usually reduction is not difficult and the following essentials must be kept firmly in mind. First, of course, be sure of the diagnosis. Second, it is most necessary to have a clear picture in mind of the exact direction that the humeral head must move in order to slide into the glenoid cavity and the third essential is not to become excited and try to hurry. Hard jerks and shotgun moves must be avoided because this will cause added damage to the tissues. Every severe joint injury is immediately followed by a spasm which contracts the surrounding muscles to protect the traumatized part and this spasm must be released before reduction of the dislocation is possible. Slow, powerful, continuous traction will tire the contracted muscles and when they release, the humeral head will slip back easily into its proper alignment.

Since heat helps to induce relaxation to the spastic muscles, it may be applied after reduction unless there is swelling from effusion, in which case an ice bag is applied. A dislocation almost always results in a tearing of the capsule and ligaments along with trauma to the rotor cuff. Occasionally all efforts by traction will fail to effect muscular relaxation in which case it must be accomplished under anaesthesia.

After reduction, the articulation must be immobilized by taping as shown in Figs. 49, 50 and 51, and treated as a severe sprain. If there is swelling, the tape strapping will be a great aid in forcing the fluid out of the tissues and it should remain in place for thirty-six to forty-eight hours. The arm must be further immobilized by the use of a sling and kept at complete rest. As stated above, an ice bag should be used during this period if effusion is present.

After forty-eight hours the tape can be removed, the muscles massaged lightly and heat may be applied. Then the shoulder should be re-taped for another forty-eight hour period. However, during this second period the patient should be instructed to begin passive exercise if the effusion has subsided. Instruct him to lean forward at the waist and slowly let the arm hang down and swing it gently in an oval arc (Fig. 136) but NEVER let it swing outward in an anterior or subglenoid dislocation. This will rotate the humeral head inward and not allow it to dislocate again, neither will it strain the injured tissues.

Prolonged immobilization may cause adhesions, ankylosis and atrophy, particularly in older persons who must be watched closely and encouraged to exercise as soon as the swelling subsides. Younger, active, supple persons are not nearly as apt to acquire a stiff shoulder after dislocation. The exercise should consist of ten or twelve oval arcs done three times a day, and except when doing this exercise, the arm should be kept in the sling, where it should remain for two to three weeks. The sling is necessary for two reasons, first, to inhibit untoward movements and second, to keep the weight of the arm from pulling down on the injured tissue.

After approximately the second week, the first exercise should be increased in intensity and the following ones added as shown in the chapter on exercises. These exercises should be continued until the maximum improvement is attained. The patient must be instructed to avoid movements that can cause a recurrence of the dislocation, such as fast outward movements that would cause external rotation, and backward reaches.

THE ACUTE ANTERIOR DISLOCATION

This is the most common of all shoulder dislocations and also the easiest to reduce. The deltoid will be spastic and difficult to indent by finger pressure. Since the deltoid is a powerful muscle and acts as a cap over the shoulder, the spasm must be overcome before reduction is possible. The patient will be in pain and will hold his arm against his body with the elbow flexed.

STEPS IN THE REDUCTION OF THE ANTERIOR DISLOCATION

1. Have the patient lie on his back on the adjusting table.

2. The doctor sits on a stool on the affected side with the median line of his body in line with the patient's shoulder.

3. The doctor removes his shoe, then grasps the patient's arm with both hands and slowly pulls the arm toward him.

4. The arch of the doctor's foot is carefully placed under the patient's armpit. If it is the right arm that is injured, the right foot is used, and vice versa for the left (Fig. 42).

5. The doctor slowly pulls the patient's arm toward him while at the same time pushing his leg away from his body, thus exerting pressure under the patient's axilla. This will produce powerful traction for release of the spasm. This steady, firm pull may have to be held for fifteen to thirty seconds before the spasm releases. Be very careful not to jerk the arm. The traction usually relieves the pain to a degree (Fig. 42).

6. Slowly rotate the humeral head inward using more pull and traction if necessary, and it is at this time that the head will usually slip into place and the movement will be distinctly felt by the doctor.

7. Take the foot from under the axilla but do not release all of the traction with the hands. Place one hand on the inside of the patient's elbow after it has been flexed; lay the other arm over the patient's forearm and wrist and with some traction on the elbow, rotate the arm inward and up on to the chest (Figs. 43 and 44). This will complete the reduction. Then have the patient hold the arm in that position with his uninjured one and immediately apply the taping as outlined in Figs. 49, 50, 51 and 53, and place the arm in a sling. It is advisable to take another x-ray to be certain that it is in its proper place. A lateral view will show it most clearly.

THE POSTERIOR DISLOCATION

The posterior dislocation does not occur nearly as frequently as does the anterior one and for that reason it may be overlooked. It occurs from a force suddenly encountered as in a blow to the anterior part of the shoulder, driving it to the posterior, or, when the force is to the arm, pulling it backward while the arm is in a state of outward rotation, allowing the head of the humerus to rotate externally, causing the head to dislocate from the posterior portion of the glenoid cavity. The history will reveal the injury followed by pain and limitation of movement, and it will appear to be deformed. When inspected from the side, the posterior area will appear fuller and the coracoid process will be very prominently felt upon palpation. The area where the humeral head is normally situated will feel and appear somewhat hollow and it will be found that the index finger can be pushed into this space to about the second joint. X-rays from an AP view may fail to show the dislocation but a lateral film will show it better.

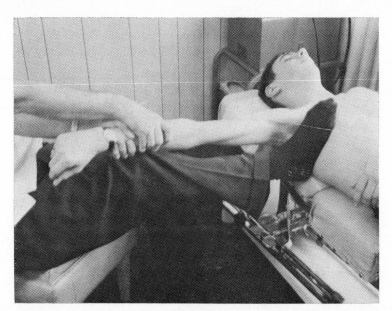

Fig. 42

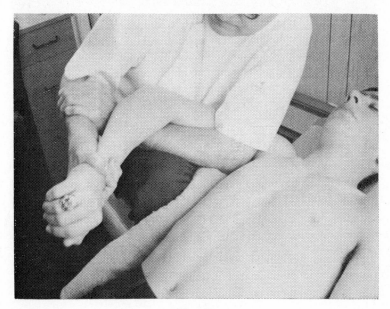

Fig. 43

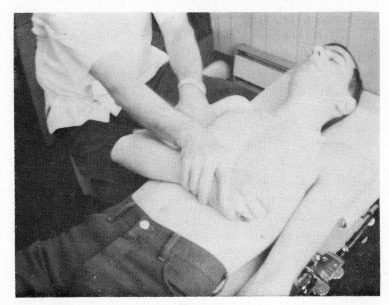

Fig. 44

STEPS IN THE REDUCTION OF THE POSTERIOR DISLOCATION

1. Have the patient sit on the adjusting table with the back of the shoulders toward the headpiece. Place two pillows on the headward end of the table.

2. The doctor then removes his shoe and sits on a stool or chair on the opposite side of the injured shoulder and places the calf of his leg upon the pillows as shown in Fig. 45.

3. Then the patient should slowly lie backward so that the lower portions of the scapulae lie across the doctor's shin.

4. The doctor then adjusts his position so that his shoulder, which is nearest the patient's head, is about in line with the patient's uninjured shoulder. If necessary for comfort, a small folded towel or foam pad may be placed over the doctor's shinbone. The doctor's left leg is used in a left dislocation and the right one in an injury on the right side.

5. The doctor then maneuvers his foot and leg so that the center part of his arch will contact the patient's affected arm below the axilla. Because of the pain, the patient will be holding his arm flexed and across his body, therefore it will be easy to grasp it above the wrist with both hands. Then the doctor, with his foot on the inside of the patient's arm, starts to push it outward while simultaneously holding the forearm firmly with his hands. The humeral head must be pushed outward slowly but with gently increasing pressure. This may take from fifteen to thirty seconds or more, depending upon the severity of the spasm. The head of the humerus will be felt to move but the pressure of the foot must be let up at this point, but now the doctor pulls the arm toward himself to complete the correction (Fig. 46). Always keep a picture in mind of the excursion that the humeral head must make, outward and around the corner and into the glenoid cavity.

6. The patient is instructed to keep the arm in this position until the tape is applied. The taping is almost the same as outlined in Figs. 49, 50 and 51, except that it is started at the back of the shoulder and pulled toward the front as shown in Fig. 54. An ice bag should be used over the tape if there is any effusion and the arm placed in a sling for two to three weeks. The program of exercises is the same as outlined in the case management of the anterior dislocation. See chapter on exercises, except in this instance, do not use those shown in Figs. 136 and 137.

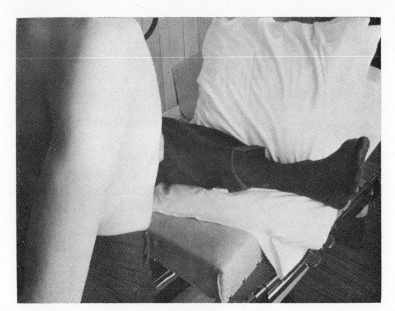

Fig. 45

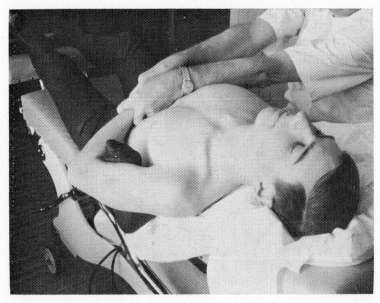

Fig. 46

The following is a case history from the writer's files which is in every way typical of the situation under discussion. The patient was a farmer who had been thrown by a horse the day before and had landed on his shoulder. When he appeared at the office the next morning he was in much pain, holding the arm closely to the front of his body with the other hand, stating that he had difficulty sleeping because of the pain. Upon inspection and palpation, the posterior fullness was noted as well as the prominent coracoid process and the hollow, soft area at the anterior. The index finger test was positive and it was diagnosed as a posterior dislocation. This was verified by x-ray which also eliminated the possbility of fracture.

The dislocation was reduced by the methods outlined above; he was taped, the arm placed in a sling and given an appointment two days later. No ice bag was advised because there was no effusion. When he returned, he stated that he was free of pain and had slept well. The tape was removed and heat applied and the muscles relaxed with fairly deep massage. Tape was re-applied, the arm was again placed in the sling and he was instructed to do the exercise as outlined and he was told to return in three days.

When he came in for that appointment he stated that he felt so good that he had been doing his work and was riding the tractor picking corn—which was strictly against the advice given him; however, he did say that he worked with the arm in the sling. This time he was not taped because of skin irritation, but was told to use the sling for two more weeks and to continue with the exercises. He was not given another appointment but a month later he returned with a painfully sprained lower back. His arm was painfree and in every respect capable of the full range of movement.

THE SUBGLENOID DISLOCATION

This is one of the most difficult of all shoulder dislocations to reduce. In the majority of cases an anaesthetic or heavy sedation should be used, usually by an orthopedic surgeon.

The humeral head drops downward from the glenoid cavity. Therefore, in order to reduce the dislocation, the head must first be drawn somewhat outward and then upward into its correct relationship with the glenoid. The writer believes that the reason this dislocation is so painful and more difficult to reduce than the other dislocations is that it does not have the powerful muscles to aid in giving the arm support. In the anterior dislocation both the deltoid and pectoralis support the head and arm. There is also muscular spasm in the subglenoid dislocation but they are not in direct contact with the head and upper part of the arm when it has been dislocated downward. Therefore, this allows more stretching and injury to the ligaments and tendons of the rotary cuff.

The writer has, on a few occasions, reduced this type of dislocation, though not with much enthusiasm, because of pain to the patient. However, since occasions do arise when it becomes a necessity, the steps will be outlined.

The patient will be in great pain, holding the injured arm flexed and close to his body, supporting it with the other hand. Upon inspection, palpation and comparison with the uninjured shoulder, a depression or hollowness will be found where the humeral head should be. The head will be found in a line downward from the acromioclavicular joint. The deltoid will be very spastic and tense. The patient should be x-rayed, preferably both shoulders for comparison.

STEPS IN THE REDUCTION OF THE SUBGLENOID DISLOCATION

1. Have the patient lie on his back on the adjusting table. If it is his right arm that is injured, then the doctor should sit so that his own left shoulder is in line with the patient's right shoulder (Figs. 47 and 48).

2. The doctor then takes a folded towel, small pillow or a piece of foam rubber and places it against the upper, lateral chest wall of the patient and then places his knee lightly on the protective pad.

3. The doctor then slips his hand and arm slowly between the patient's body and flexed elbow, then grasps his own arm with his other hand thus encircling the patient's arm with his arms. He then gradually slides his own arms upward on the patient's arm while his knee exerts firm pressure on the patient's body through the protective rib pad (Fig. 47).

4. The doctor then pulls the patient's arm slowly and somewhat outward from the body while at the same time pushing inward with this knee to stabilize the patient. In this way traction is produced to relax the muscles. As the arm moves away from the patient's body, the direction of pull is changed and the arm is pulled slowly upward as shown in Fig. 48. The patient's forearm has remained flexed during this entire procedure. Never use any quick movements or jerks since

136

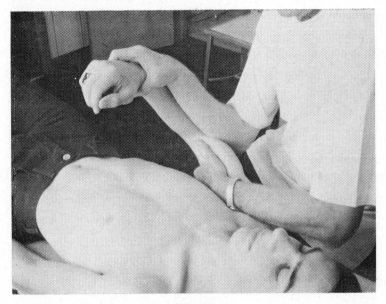

Fig. 47

The above picture is shown ONLY for reasons of clarity so that the knee contact and the exact position of the doctor's arms as they encircle the patient's arm can be illustrated. In an actual subglenoid dislocation it would be impractical because of pain, and therefore inadvisable to move the injured arm this far from the patient's body.

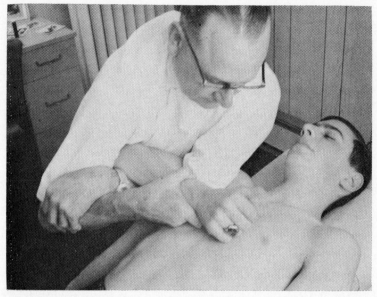

Fig. 48

Note how close the doctor's arms are to the patient's body. This is the actual positioning used in the reduction. The patient's injured arm is in the doctor's axilla and the distal portion of the doctor's humerus is just below the head of the patient's dislocated humerus. With this contact, the doctor has perfect control over the patient's arm because he can pull outward, hold and, with the thrust of his body, move the arm upward near its normal position.

the pain is severe enough even with the most careful manipulation. The humerus can be felt sliding into place. The patient is told to hold the arm in position with the other hand and is helped to a sitting position for the taping.

5. The taping is the same as outline in Figs. 49, 50 and 51, with two exceptions. The first strips of tape are pulled upward and over the deltoid covering it as shown in Figs. 50 and a piece or two of tape may be brought under the elbow and over the shoulder as in the acromioclavicular taping shown in Fig. 35. The arm is then placed in a sling for a month to six weeks, a much longer healing period than is needed for the other dislocations discussed.

6. Exercises. These patients should be checked every few days and as soon as feasible the doctor should start the exercises. Instruct the patient to lie on his back on the bed with his head at the foot end because the headboard would be in the way for the exercises (Figs. 134 and 135). First the arm is raised straight up and rotated INWARD. When that can be accomplished, the arm should also be raised over the head so it comes to rest above the head in a straight line with the body. When these exercises can readily be done, the following one is added: sit in front of a closed door so that the injured arm is in a straight line with the knob. Grasp the knob with the hand and slowly lean back so the muscles are stretched. Continue the exercises until free movement has been restored.

TAPING USED IN SHOULDER DISLOCATIONS

The pull or tension applied to the adhesive during the taping procedure is very important. In an anterior dislocation, the doctor pulls the tape from front to back and in the posterior dislocation it is from back to front.

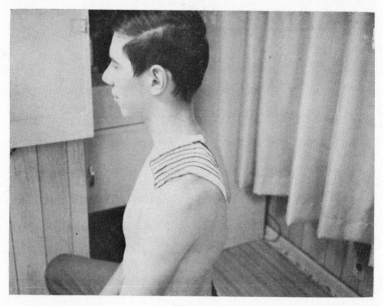

Fig. 49

The photograph above shows the first step in a shoulder taping. Tear the strips of tape long enough so that they extend down the chest about as far as shown and down the back to a point about three inches below the superior border of the scapula. Six to eight strips will be needed.

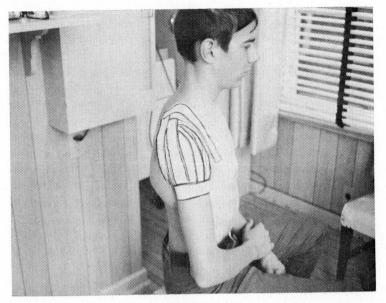

Fig. 50

In the second step in all shoulder tapings the pull of the tape is upward as shown in Fig. 52 EXCEPT in acromio-clavicular situations where the pull is downward. From eight to ten strips will be needed and all are applied with the upward pull. The anchor strip is the one that is closest to the neck and the one that APPEARS to encircle the arm. It does NOT encircle and is placed to anchor and cover the ends of the perpendicular strips.

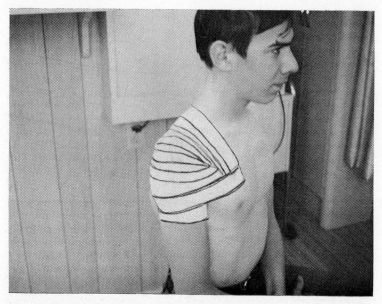

Fig. 51

The third layer is applied with a pushing pressure directed against the arm as well as slightly upward. The strips are torn long enough so they will cover the chest wall as shown and also the greater portion of the scapula as shown in Fig. 33. Depending upon the size of the patient, from ten to fourteen strips will be needed.

The doctor holds the tape horizontally, one end in each hand, grasped so that the fingertips touch the adhesive side and the base of his thumb contacts the non-adhesive side. He then places the center of the length of the tape against the center of the arm (center when judged from anterior to posterior) about an inch or two below the deltoid. He then pushes against the arm and at the same time also pushes slightly upward so that when the tape ends are in place, they are higher than the center starting point. This will form a wide U shape as shown. Each succeeding strip is placed a little higher than the preceding one until the shoulder area is covered as shown.

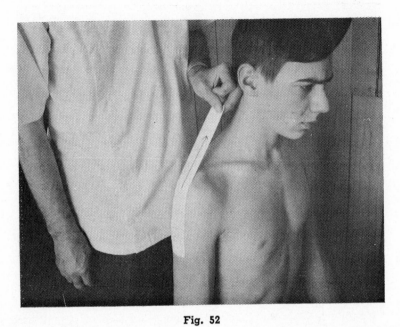

Fig. 52

The direction of pull in all shoulder tapings is upward as shown, EX-
CEPT in acromio-clavicular lesions where the pull is DOWNWARD.

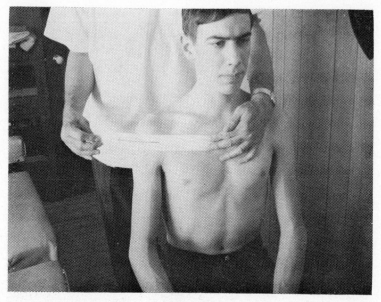

Fig. 53

This picture shows the direction of tension or direction of pull used in applying tape in an anterior dislocation of the shoulder and in a lesion of the long head of the biceps tendon. In all taping procedures, the doctor must always have in mind the direction in which the joint migrated and apply tape pressure in the opposite direction.

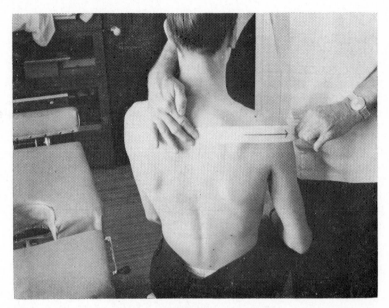

Fig. 54

This photograph shows the direction of pull when taping a posterior dislocation.

THE RECURRENT DISLOCATION

In this situation the humeral head will migrate either to the anterior, posterior or to the subglenoid area, however, it will almost always follow the pattern of the initial dislocation. The danger in any dislocation is the possibility of its becoming recurrent and this is especially applicable to the shoulder joint because of its wide range of movement and exposure to blows, falls, stresses and strains.

An individual's age, activity and occupation should all be taken into consideration before any radical measures are advised. For example, a sedentary worker who is not active in sports should not worry too much about a shoulder that becomes troublesome once a year. The real handicap of recurring dislocations are to those persons who are in occupations such as farming, mechanics, building trades or are active amateur or professional athletes.

Recurrent dislocations begin, of course, with a violent accident, such as a fall from a piece of machinery or a tumble down a flight of stairs. Later, much less force is needed to produce a subsequent dislocation and after a number of them have occurred, the integrity of the articulation can become so weakened that even combing the hair or reaching back for a billfold is sufficient to cause the head to slip out of the glenoid cavity. When that point is reached, the patient should be advised to have surgical assistance.

The writer had an interesting case depicting the progression in this type of lesion. A sixteen year old high school girl was afflicted with epilepsy and while in a seizure, would frequently fall. The first dislocation in her shoulder resulted from a fall down a flight of stairs while in a seizure. The writer was called to the house where the girl was crying from pain and holding her arm in the typical manner.

The dislocation was to the anterior with no fracture. The head of the humerus, upon palpation and inspection, was found to be approximately two and one half inches removed from the glenoid. By placing a chair and sitting beside the bed, the reduction was accomplished by the method outlined under anterior dislocations. The taping was applied as described, the arm placed in a sling and the father advised to bring the girl in to check the humeral position by x-ray. She was checked at intervals and apparent normal healing took place and she had no difficulty for six months.

Then, during another seizure, she fell on the floor, dislocating the same shoulder in the same way for the second time. Again the

146

writer was called and the same corrective measures and case management procedures were followed and once more there was apparent recovery. However, over a period of three or four months, the arm was twice more dislocated. Finally the girl would lie down when she felt that an attack was imminent but by that time the muscle spasms created by the seizures were sufficient to cause dislocation. It was at this point that the writer advised surgical intervention for the purpose of shortening the overstretched tendons and ligaments.

THE OLD OR CHRONIC DISLOCATION

The old or chronic dislocations can be classified into two types:
1. THE NEGLECTED DISLOCATION is the one that has no professional care at the time of injury, is neglected by the individual and is self-diagnosed as a sprain and treated as such.

2. THE UNRECOGNIZED DISLOCATION is the one that is missed by the doctor. When the patient comes for relief, he does not x-ray or make a careful examination and fails to locate the difficulty telling the patient that it is only a bad sprain and advises rest and heat.

In either event, the patient will come in complaining of pain and limitation of movement that is becoming progressively worse. Examination will reveal that the shoulder is stiff and both active and passive movements are grossly inhibited. The patient will give information of an accident some weeks or a few months previously and will state that he is very concerned regarding the pain and limitation of movement. X-rays should be taken and a thorough examination be made to locate the exact cause of the difficulty. When a dislocation is present and the humeral head has been out of the glenoid cavity for weeks or months, the soft tissue may become adherent and the head may have become adhesed to its place of dislocation, thus making reduction difficult at best and impossible at worst. Therefore, if reduction is attempted, forceful moves should NEVER be used.

The most frequent of the two dislocations just described is the anterior and the posterior is next. Though the posterior occurs less frequently, it is also the most overlooked of the three possible dislocations. The subglenoid is not only more painful but also the most apparent since it does not have the heavy muscles to hide its position and therefore can hardly be missed.

While it is true that many of these chronic dislocations will require surgical intervention, there is still a fair percentage that can be reduced if the fixation is not too severe. First, determine the amount of movement remaining in the arm without binding or pain. Next, ascertain the patient's pain tolerance by moving the arm beyond his own scope of movement. Then gently try the corrective moves. If the patient does not seem too uncomfortable then try to make the correction but always remembering not to use any forceful pulling and jerking which could do harm. Just use the steady, slow, progressive pull.

The writer's files contain a case which illustrates this situation clearly. The patient was a thirty-eight year old farmer, in good health and with very well developed chest and deltoid muscles. Seven weeks before coming to the office, while riding a tractor through the field, he also pulled corn stalks with the tractor moving. Once, when reaching back for a stalk, it didn't give, but his shoulder did. He said that he felt something move and there was a sharp pain. As is so often the case, he made his own diagnosis and thought that it was either a sprain or pulled muscle. Though the shoulder was quite painful, he nevertheless continued working, even though he was unable to raise the arm. But, being an ambitious person, he still did not seek help because he found that he could ride the tractor, steering it with the right hand, and give the left arm some protection by keeping it inside his coat. After a few more weeks even this doughty individual had to give up and seek help when the pain became intense and the arm useless.

The shoulder was carefully examined and x-rayed and a posterior dislocation was clearly apparent. It was explained to him that because of the seven week time lapse, there would no doubt be a fixation of the humeral head in the soft tissues and that surgery would possibly be necessary, and at this point he called his wife to the office. The writer told them that he would try reduction but gave no encouragement as to the results. After a short, private discussion, they agreed to try the chiropractic way first.

The patient was placed on the adjusting table and treated as outlined for the posterior correction on page 133. Traction was used in gradually increasing intensity for about thirty seconds when the humeral head moved outward with very little pain and slowly pulled into the socket. He was taped as directed on pages 140, 141 and 142, the arm put in a sling and he was told to return in two days. When he returned, there was much improvement and he had but little pain. The tape was removed, the shoulder massaged to loosen the muscles and the same adjustment given, but MUCH milder traction used. This was done because the tissues needed some stretching and also because there was a possibility that a posterior subluxation would follow the direction of the dislocation. He was then re-taped, the arm replaced in the sling and he was told to return in three days.

When he came for his third appointment, the same procedure was followed as that described in the second visit, except he was not taped, and the exercises were begun. In a chronic situation, the exercises are started a bit later than in the acute injury. When he returned a week later for his last appointment, he was entirely free of pain and had normal arm and shoulder movement. He was advised to increase the intensity of the exercises and to continue with the sling for three weeks. This patient received a total of four adjustments and this, along with proper case management, produced for him a completely normal arm and shoulder.

In all dislocations, and particularly the chronic type, it is advisable to give a complete chiropractic adjustment, giving special attention to the cervical and upper dorsal areas and the first rib because the strain put on the other groups of muscles and the tension produced by the pain will have a tendency to cause subluxations.

The above described patient has had no further difficulty with that shoulder in the twelve years that have since passed. Four years ago he injured the right shoulder and lost no time in having it checked. That, however, proved to be a severe sprain from which he rapidly recovered. This man's first shoulder injury made very good chiropractic patients of the entire family and produced many referrals, and to this day the family has regular chiropractic care. We, as a profession, should realize the importance of proper articular care—it is a splendid practice builder.

A CASE HISTORY OF THE UNREDUCED DISLOCATION

This was the case of a housewife, age 65, and very obese, about 245 pounds. Three months previous to examination in the office, she had slipped on icy steps coming out of church. She had grasped the railing to protect against a fall, thus twisting and pulling on the shoulder joint with her great weight, causing the humeral head to be forced away from the glenoid. The pain was immediate and intense and movement restricted at once. She was rushed to a medical doctor who diagnosed it as a dislocation. She was given a strong sedative and, according to the patient, he twisted it around a few times and then told her that it was in place. No x-rays were taken before or after the treatment. Her arm was placed in a sling and she was given pain pills.

Since she had almost no relief, she returned several times complaining of the pain but was told that it would take time to get well. Discouraged, she decided to go to an osteopath. This doctor again did not x-ray the shoulder but used manipulation and told her that it was in place. Still with no relief, her family decided to take her to their chiropractic doctor. This doctor, from another state, called the writer and made an appointment for a consultation since he did not care to take the case after learning of the history.

When the patient came to our office she was holding the arm with the other hand and, when sitting, would place the elbow on her lap for support. She could not raise the arm without the aid of the other hand and movement was extremely limited even with the help of the other arm.

Upon inspection and palpation the writer suspected a subglenoid dislocation and x-rays were taken which verified the diagnosis. It was the worst dislocation ever encountered by the writer, the humeral head being four and one-half inches from the glenoid cavity, and no attempt was made to reduce it because of the length of time involved. Instead she was advised to have surgical correction. Since she lived in close proximity to Minneapolis, she had it done there. Four months later her son wrote, stating that his mother's arm was almost well and thanked our office for locating the problem and giving the correct advice. Again, the writer wishes to emphasize the necessity of a correct diagnosis, confirmed by x-ray if at all possible, and the importance of proper advice in these types of cases.

The most interesting and unusual case of shoulder dislocation in the writer's thirty-six years of practice was that of a child with both shoulders dislocated anteriorly. This was an eight month old girl who had been a very difficult delivery because she weighed fifteen and one-half pounds at birth. The child cried excessively and the parents noticed that she did not use her arms as other children of that age do. Several times they took her to the medical doctor who had delivered her and were told that there was nothing really wrong and that she would outgrow it. The mother was nonetheless very concerned and brought her to our office. She told of the difficult delivery with instruments, which, in her opinion, had been unusually rough. This was her fourth child and all had been very large babies but none of the others had received birth injuries and her mother's instinct told her that something was very amiss with this child.

In examining the infant, it was noted that she held her arms tightly to her sides. Upon trying to move the arms outward and upward, she would cry violently and her face became contorted, definitely registering extreme pain. X-rays were made which showed that both shoulders were completely dislocated anteriorly. After a consultation with Dr. Myrna Schultz, we decided to try to reduce the dislocations. Dr. Myrna stood at the side of the baby, who had been placed on her back on a pillow on the adjusting table, holding the baby's body and gently pulling toward her. The writer stood on the other side of the table, placed the palm of one hand under the child's armpit and with the other hand, grasped the arm. The slow, careful, directional pull was used as described in the anterior dislocation. The baby understandably screamed both from fright and pain. The mother cried and promptly fainted. Dr. Myrna had to attend to the mother while the writer completed the reductions in both shoulders. The baby's arms were then bound by wrapping the arms and body with two ace bandages taped together lengthwise, forming one very long bandage.

Method: Encircle one arm, not too tightly, go around the body, encircle the other arm, again go around the body, back to the first arm and repeat in this manner to the end of the bandage, anchoring it with tape. The child was treated in this manner once a week for six weeks, each time showing less and less pain for the baby. The mother was instructed in the proper method of exercising the child's arms and at the end of the period of care, the child had full and normal use of both arms. A few years ago the mother sent us a picture of this girl in the act of going through her cheerleading routines at high school.

The following is a summary of the steps to be particularly remembered when caring for dislocations:

1. Take a complete case history, noting when and how the injury occurred. Also note the type of accident and if it was a fall, have the patient describe how he fell so that the doctor can deduce reasonably well whether the main force was to the hand, elbow or shoulder area.

2. Inspect, palpate and compare with the normal shoulder. If at all possible, use x-rays to confirm or eliminate the presence of fractures and locate the exact direction of the dislocation. Both shoulders should be x-rayed so that abnormalities in the injured one can be more easily discerned.

3. The doctor must know exactly what he is going to do, and if necessary, think the procedure through for a minute or two so that he can be sure. Then he must get the patient, as well as himself, situated in the correct positions before any reduction is begun, and he must remember never to hurry or become excited.

4. The spasm must be relaxed before a successful reduction can be accomplished, therefore slow, strong and gradually increasing traction must be used. This may become tiring to the doctor before the spasms will release and ten seconds will seem more like thirty or forty.

5. After the reduction is accomplished, the correct case management procedures must be used as outlined, both the taping and sling support.

6. Exercises are extremely important and cannot be neglected. The patient must be instructed in which ones to do and it must be made plain to him that he is responsible for this part of his recovery. It must be explained to him that the exercises are for the purpose of strengthening the muscles, avoiding adhesions which will cause future trouble and possibly surgery, and to restore to him a normal shoulder without the prospect of future recurring dislocations. The patient most certainly wants a normal shoulder but it is remarkable how many will neglect the exercises unless their importance is clearly defined and stressed.

THE SUBLUXATION OF THE SHOULDER JOINT

This is a more common lesion than has been appreciated by the chiropractic profession as a whole. It is comparable to the irritation and erosion of the semilunars produced by a subluxated tibia which results in a painful and unstable knee, frequently accompanied by arthritis. These situations can be corrected and prevented by locating and adjusting the subluxation. The shoulder, because of its wide range of movement, its vulnerability to falls, blows and occupational strains, may become subluxated very easily.

It is the writer's opinion that such common ailments of the shoulder as degenerative tendonitis, subacromial bursitis, or subdeltoid bursitis, supraspinatous bursitis and bicipital lesions may be caused, in a great number of cases, by the so often overlooked shoulder subluxation. Since all of these structures are intimate with the glenohumeral joint and work in unison with it, it is logical to assume that a subluxation of the head of the humerus with the glenoid cavity can irritate and cause a wearing and weakening of these structures, since all authorities agree that these syndroms are of a non-bacterial and non-infectious origin. The cause and progression of these conditions is strictly mechanical.

All articulations have a weak spot. In the knee it is the menisci; in the shoulder it is the musculocutaneous cuff and the biceps tendon. The glenoid labrum, by its position of attachment around the margin of the glenoid cavity, is especially exposed to erosion which can lead to an unstable head which, in turn, will be followed by strain, irritation and a weakening of the related tissues.

The shoulder joint may become subluxated in four directions, therefore, after a dislocation, it is always advisable to check the shoulder periodically for at least two months because, after severe trauma, the integrity of the surrounding tissues may be weakened which, in turn, would allow the humeral head to subluxate in the same directional pathway as the earlier dislocation.

It is not difficult to visualize how a subluxation of the shoulder joint, over a period of time, could have an adverse effect and be the underlying cause in the rupture of the rotor cuff tendons. The reason for most of these ruptures is wear and tear degeneration caused by an abnomal mechanical process, namely the subluxation.

The middle aged working man is the one who most often appears with a cuff rupture. He may have no history of severe, traumatic injury. Rather, upon questioning, he will state that he had a small bump to the shoulder, or he made an awkward reach, or that his shoulder had been uncomfortable off and on over the past several months and now suddenly became severely painful. When a patient makes statements similar to the above mentioned, the doctor can be quite certain that he is dealing with a long standing subluxation involving wear and tear degeneration. In ruptures caused by severe trauma there is seldom a degenerative process with which to reckon.

The tendon of the supraspinatous is also bound to be affected by a shoulder subluxation because of its location, contact and function. Its function is to stabilize the humeral head in the glenoid cavity during all of its movements. Any misalignment of the head could greatly affect the tendon and cause irritation and tendinitis.

The long head of the biceps is intimately related to the shoulder joint and is affected by all movements of the humeral head and glenoid cavity. In addition, it has the specific duty of anchoring this powerful muscle. Many times there is the added complication of bursitis since it is logical for the bursa to become involved whenever there is irritation in the surrounding shoulder structures. The shoulder subluxation, if accompanied by bursitis, should not be corrected until after the acute stage has subsided. It is also not advisable to attempt correction after the rupture of the rotator cuff.

It is the writer's contention that the shoulder joint be given thorough attention after any injury, no matter how trivial it may seem. In our office, every shoulder injury or complaint of discomfort is checked for a possible subluxation as well as spinal and rib subluxations. The writer has found and corrected many hundreds of these situations and feels that it is an important phase because it prevents many serious future shoulder syndromes.

I. The Superior Shoulder Subluxation

The most often overlooked and the most frequent subluxation of the shoulder is the superior one which occurs when the arm is used to break a fall and the head of the humerus is driven upward. Since the joint is protected by an arch formed by the coracoid process, the acromion and the coracoacromial ligament, it is practically impossible for a dislocation to occur to the superior unless there is a fracture and torn ligaments of the arch structure. Because of the protective arch, it is impossible to palpate superior misalignments of the humeral head but x-rays will show the subluxation very clearly provided that comparative films are made of both shoulders.

ADJUSTMENT OF THE SUPERIOR SUBLUXATION

1. Have the patient lie on his back on the adjusting table. The doctor should sit on the side of the subluxation with his body turned toward the shoulder. The center of the crest of the doctor's ilium should be in line with the patient's knee joint (Fig. 55).

2. The doctor then removes his shoe, grasps the patient's arm and places the anterior portion of his heel under the patient's armpit. The right foot is used when adjusting the right arm and vice versa.

3. Since there is no spasm, there is no need to hold traction. With the doctor's foot under the axilla, he pulls on the arm to produce moderate traction. Then he rotates the patient's arm inward and gives a short, snappy move towards his own body (Fig. 55).

154

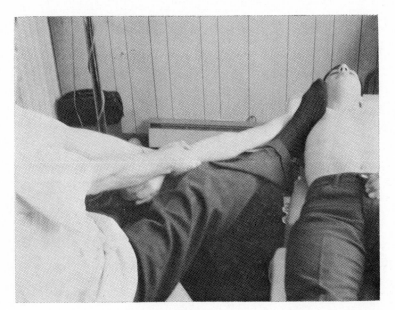

Fig. 55

There are other contacts and moves that can be used to correct a superior shoulder subluxation, however, the above outlined is not only effective, but safe since the doctor's foot acts as a deterrent against sprain or dislocation of the humeral head to the inferior.

The doctor will have to use his own judgment concerning the necessity of taping after this correction. In some cases it is advisable to do so and, when necessary, use the taping procedure outlined for a dislocation. The writer has corrected many where tape was not used. The patients received immediate, marked relief and their shoulders were normal in just a very few adjustments.

II. The Anterior Shoulder Subluxation

The anterior subluxation is second in order of frequency and is relatively easy to locate. Many times the cause of it is an accident where the arm was used for protection in breaking a fall. It may also happen when pulling or lifting a heavy object, particularly if the person slips or gets off balance. This misalignment can be detected after almost any anterior dislocation. Very often dislocations are thought to be completely reduced yet the shoulder is not normal and it is this subluxation that must be corrected before the patient is pain free.

The writer particularly remembers one case that made him decide to check all shoulders for subluxations when the history showed an accident, no matter how long ago. This patient, a thirty year old man, came in about twenty-five years ago. He was a truck driver who had fallen from his truck and had landed on his arm. Since he was delivering oxygen to the hospital, he was immediately taken in and x-rayed. The film showed a complete anterior dislocation of the right shoulder. The orthopedic surgeon reduced the dislocation and used the usual supportive measures.

After four months had elapsed, the man still could not raise the arm overhead and he stated that the shoulder had a constant gnawing ache. He came to our office asking to be examined and to find out whether or not chiropractic could help him. The subluxation was very apparent and quickly adjusted. Since he lived quite some distance away, he was given an appointment in a week at which time he was again scheduled to deliver oxygen to the hospital on his route. When he appeared for that appointment he was a very happy person since all pain had disappeared and he had complete and normal motion of the entire shoulder. When he left he kept asking, "Why didn't THEY find it?" Needless to say, this case was responsible for a great number of referred patients.

156

PROCEDURE IN LOCATING THE ANTERIOR SUBLUXATION

This is the easiest of all the shoulder subluxations to palpate, locate and compare with the normal one. In many instances it can be located visually since the area appears fuller than the normal one. Palpation will elicit tenderness. It is advisable to palpate both shoulders simultaneously in order to quickly locate the differences in them. The subluxated one will have taut and stringy muscular fibers over it (Fig. 56). In palpation, the coracoid process must not be confused with the humeral head. It—the coracoid process—will feel prominent and many times may be tender because the muscles may also be painful and under strain because of the irritation caused by the subluxated head. The coracoid is slightly higher than the humeral head.

ADJUSTMENT OF THE ANTERIOR SHOULDER SUBLUXATION

In this correction, three different methods will be shown.

MOVE I:

The patient should sit on the palpation stool and the doctor should stand behind him. The patient is then instructed to raise his arm parallel with the floor and to place the palm of his hand behind his neck. If it is the right shoulder that is to be corrected, the right palm is placed on the back of the right side of the neck.

The doctor places both arms in front of the patient and interlocks his fingers telling the patient to drop his elbow into the doctor's hands. The doctor's body is in the center of the patient's spinal area. It is best if the doctor's body does not contact either of the patient's scapulae.

The doctor then tells the patient to relax the arm and drop its weight into the doctor's hands. The doctor then gives a short, snappy pull straight toward his own body. Usually the movement will definitely be felt and often the "pop" will be heard as the humerus glides back into position (Fig. 57). See Note, Fig. 57.

MOVE II:

The position of the patient and doctor is the same as in the foregoing one EXCEPT the patient places the palm of his hand on the opposite side of the neck. If it is the right shoulder to be adjusted, the patient places the right palm against the back left side of his neck (Fig. 58). This is done because sometimes the position in Move I is not quite comfortable to the patient and by changing

157

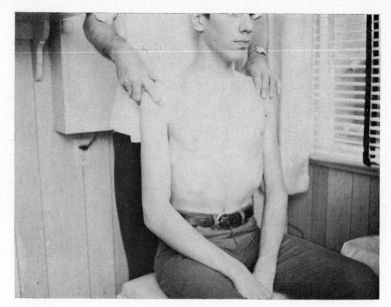

Fig. 56

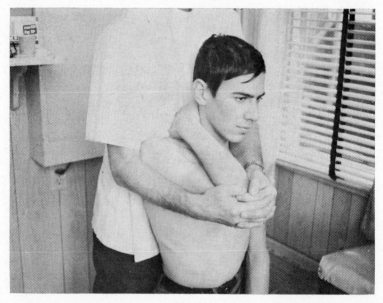

Fig. 57

Note: Do NOT use the moves shown in Figs. 57 and 58 on old or fragile persons. Use instead the one shown in Fig. 59, **lightly.**

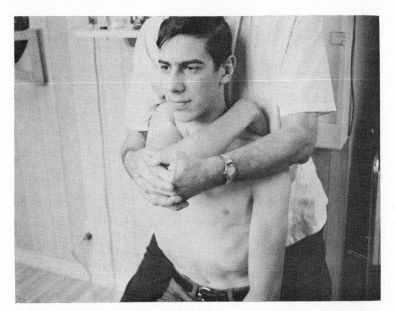

Fig. 58

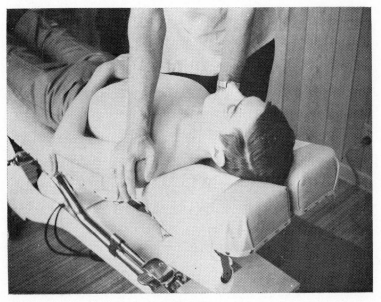

Fig. 59

to this position the head of the humerus is rotated inward. The patient is more relaxed and the humeral head in good position for the corrective move. See Note under Fig. 57.

It is the writer's opinion that at times the head is not directly anteriorly subluxated but is rotated inward to some degree, therefore, the different position allows a better and less painful correction. The doctor should have the patient try both positions and use the one that is most comfortable.

MOVE III:

Many times in the acute shoulder sprain there is also an anterior subluxation and it may be so painful that the arm cannot be raised parallel to the floor. When this is the situation, the patient is placed on his back on the adjusting table with both arms folded across the waistline. The doctor stands on the opposite side of injury and places the palm of his hand on the injured shoulder in such a manner that the thumb portion is over the subluxated humeral head. The doctor's other hand is placed in the same position on the uninjured shoulder for the purpose of stabilizing the patient when the thrust is given (Fig. 59). The doctor then gives a short, snappy thrust on the head of the subluxated humerus. It is advisable to check this type of injury about once a week for a month or so. See Note under Fig. 57.

III. The Posterior Subluxation

This subluxation exists more frequently than is generally realized for the reason that it is impossible to palpate and therefore difficult to locate. It can only be found through the use of comparative x-rays.

The adjustment is practically the same as that shown in Fig. 46 for the posterior dislocation EXCEPT that the outward pressure of the doctor's foot on the humerus is less because the humeral head does not need to be moved from the back of the glenoid cavity. However, MODERATE outward pressure must be applied before the pull is given on the patient's arm because the head does have to be moved away from the glenoid rim so that there will be no injury to the glenoid labrum.

IV. The Inferior Subluxation

This situation does not occur very frequently and is best determined by the use of comparative x-rays.

CORRECTION OF THE INFERIOR SUBLUXATION

For this correction, use the same contact as shown in Fig. 48 EXCEPT the thrust is given straight upward in a short, fast move. This subluxation is quite rare and usually will be encountered only in those persons who have a history of a previous subglenoid dislocation.

BRACHIAL PLEXUS PAIN

Brachial plexus pain may be a symptom or reflex pain from a visceral disease process and a careful study must be made to localize its source. Therefore, a snap diagnosis of brachial neuralgia or brachial neuritis should be avoided until the source of the pain has been determined.

Among the common conditions which are local and cause a direct irritation to the nerve components of the brachial plexus are: osteoarthritis of the cervical spine, subluxations of the cervical vertebrae with a narrowing of the intervertebral foramina, degenerative thinning of the vertebral discs, root compression by a protruding cervical disc and the scalene anticus syndrome.

It is thought by many authorities that primary brachial neuritis is rare and the term has been used to cover a lack of more precise knowledge. Brachial neuralgia or neuritis of the brachial plexus is not uncommon as a result of diabetes, trauma, toxic absorption from acute infection and malignant infiltration.

The best differentiation on the causes of brachial pain developing in the course of the brachial plexus or from conditions which simulate brachial plexus pain is outlined and grouped in the book, "Pain Syndromes," written by Judovitch and Bates. This grouping is made up by the Department of Neurology, Graduate School, University of Pennsylvania, as follows:

1. LOCAL PROCESSES. In bones, joints, ligaments, bursae, muscles and tendons, due to trauma, infection, neoplasm and metabolic disturbances. Bursitis, cervical rib, scalenus syndrome and infraspinatus syndrome. Epicondylitis, glomus tumor, muscle spasm due to early Parkinson's disease.

2. VASCULAR DISEASE. Raynaud's, Buerger's, phlebitis, aneurysm, arteritis, scalenus anticus syndrome, costoclavicular syndrome.

3. PERIPHERAL NERVE DISEASE. Neuritis, reflex dystrophies, osteoporosis, multiple and localized. Neuralgia. Role of focal

161

infections and deficiency states. Tumors and traumatic factors.

4. BRACHIAL PLEXUS DISEASE. Trauma. Tumors and other compressive factors. Cervical rib. Scalenus anticus syndrome. Superior sulcus tumor.

5. ROOT AFFECTIONS.
   (a) Inflammatory lesions. Syphilis. Suppurative and nonsuppurative processes. Herpes zoster.
   (b) Compressive lesions, in the intervertebral foramina and the epidural, subdural and subarachnoid spaces. Primary and secondary tumors and lymphoblastomas. Syphilis, tuberculosis, arachnoiditis, herniation of nucleus pulposus, chronic epidural infections, arthritis and trauma.

6. INTRAMEDULLARY SPINAL CORD LESIONS. Tumors, syringomyelia and other "central" pains.

7. REFERRED PAIN.
   (a) From the heart and great vessels
   (b) From the lungs
   (c) From the mediastinum
   (d) From the diaphragm
   (e) From the abdominal viscera
      (1) Into the left shoulder from splenic injury, pancreatitis or pancreatic carcinoma, and ruptured peptic ulcer.
      (2) Into the right shoulder from the gall bladder and liver disease, subdiaphragmatic abscess, and ruptured peptic ulcer.

8. PSYCHALGIA. The diagnostic procedures may be outlined as follows:

   1. HISTORY: Duration of pain and of associated symptoms. Character of pain and aggravating and relieving factors. Distribution of pain—local, peripheral or radicular. Weight loss and other somatic factors.

   2. OBJECTIVE EXAMINATION: Complete somatic and detailed neurological study.
      (a) Range of joint motion. Compression and traction maneuvers of cervical spine
      (b) Weakness, tone, atrophy and fibrillations

162

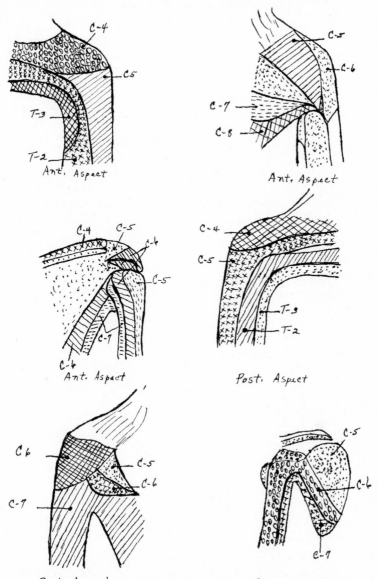

Comparison of segmental and superficial innervation of skin and deep structures of the shoulder. (Inman and Saunders)

Fig. 60

(c) Reflex changes, anesthesia, tenderness
(d) Skin temperature and color
(e) Arterial pulsations

3. ROUTINE STUDIES. Temperature range, x-ray examination of the cervical and dorsal vertebrae, the chest, the shoulder joint and scapula, urinalysis, complete blood count, blood sugar, urea nitrogen and uric acid, serologic studies and sedimentation rate.

4. SPECIAL STUDIES. Bence-Jones, basal metabolic studies, phosphatase studies, biopsy, sternal puncture, cultures. Spinal tap for hydrodynamics and detailed study of the spinal fluid. Myelogram.

5. REPEATED STUDIES. At times, repeated physical and neurological and laboratory studies are necessary.

Chapter IX

THE RIBS

SUBLUXATIONS OF THE RIBS

Subluxations of the ribs are, to a certain degree, the cause of a number of disorders and enter into the pain and discomfort pattern in many cases of shoulder and arm syndromes. These are: intercostal neuralgia, shingles, symptoms of seeming heart trouble when the subluxations are on the left side, chest pain in general and pleurisy. In many female patients rib subluxations can cause pain, swelling and lumps in the breast, causing the usual fear and worry of cancer. It is not the writer's intention to state that cancer can be cured by simply adjusting the ribs, but it IS true that many of these patients have symptoms similar to those of the dread disease and by locating these subluxated ribs and adjusting their misalignment along with the subluxated vertebrae, these symptoms will disappear if it is not cancer.

The first rib is the one that is most frequently subluxated. Next in order is the fourth, then the second, fifth and sixth. The other ribs may also become subluxated, but not nearly as frequently because they do not seem to come under the same occupational, postural or traumatic stresses as do those that are mentioned above. It must also be kept in mind that the ribs can also subluxate in their relationship with the sternum. The writer will endeavor to go thoroughly into the adjustment of the ribs, the symptoms that may result from their misalignment and the results that may be expected from the corrections. In order to do this it would be best to review the ribs and their relationship with the vertebrae and other structures with which they are intimately associated.

THE RIBS

The first seven ribs are connected behind with the vertebral column and in front through the intervention of the costal cartilages with the sternum. These ribs are called the true or vertebral-sternal ribs. The remaining five are called the false ribs, and the first three of these have their cartilages attached to the cartilages of the rib above (vertebro-chondral). The last two are free at their anterior extremities and are termed floating or vertebral ribs. The ribs vary in their direction, the upper ones being less oblique than the lower. The obliquity reaches its maximum at the ninth rib and gradually decreases from that rib to the twelfth.

The first, second, tenth, eleventh and twelfth ribs present cer-

165

tain variations from the others and are known as peculiar ribs. The first is the most curved and the shortest of all ribs. It is broad and flat, its surface looking upward and downward and its borders inward and outward. The head is small, rounded and possesses only a single articular facet, for articulation with the body of the first thoracic vertebra. The neck is narrow and rounded, the tubercle thick and prominent. There is no angle at the tubercle, but the rib is slightly bent downward at this area so that the head of the bone is directed downward. The upper body surface is marked by two shallow grooves, the grooves being separated from each other by a slight ridge, the scalene tubercle, for the attachment of the scalene anterior muscle. The anterior groove transmits the subclavian vein, the posterior groove the subclavian artery and the lowest trunk of the brachial plexus. Behind the posterior groove is a rough area for the attachment of the scalene medius muscle. The anterior border is convex, thick and rounded and its posterior part gives attachment to the first digitation of the serratus anterior. The inner border is concave and at about its center is marked by the scalene tubercle. The anterior extremity is larger and thicker than any of the other ribs.

THE SECOND RIB

This one is much longer than the first but has a very similar curvature. Its external surface is convex and looks upward and a little downward. Near the middle of it there is a rough eminence for the origin of the lower part of the serratus anterior muscle. Behind and above this is attached the scalenus posterior.

The second rib articulates with the lower portion of the body of the first dorsal and the transverse of the second dorsal vertebra. All of the rest of the ribs have the same association with the vertebra above and the one below. The first, tenth, eleventh and twelfth ribs have only a single articular facet on the head and only contacts the vertebral body in one area.

COSTOVERTEBRAL ARTICULATION

The articulations of the ribs with the vertebral column may be divided into two sets, one connecting the heads of the ribs with the bodies of the vertebrae and another uniting the necks and tubercles of the ribs with the transverse processes.

1. ARTICULATIONS OF THE HEAD OF THE RIBS

These constitute a series of gliding or arthrodial joints formed by the articulation of the heads of the typical ribs with the facets on the contiguous margins of the bodies of the thoracic vertebrae and the intervertebral fibrocartilages between them. The ligaments are:

a. the articular capsule

b. the radiate

c. the interarticular cartilage which connects the rib to the inter vertebral cartilage

2. THE COSTOTRANSVERSE ARTICULATIONS

The articular portion of the tubercle of the rib forms, with the articular surface on the adjacent transverse process, an arthrodial joint. In the eleventh and twelfth rib area this articulation is wanting. The ligaments of this joint are:

a. The articular capsule

b. The anterior costotransverse

c. The ligament of the neck of the rib

d. The ligament of the tubercles of the rib

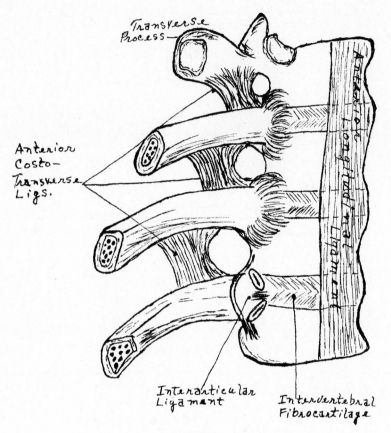

Transverse Process

Anterior Costo-Transverse Ligs.

Anterior longitudinal Ligament

Interarticular Ligamant

Intervertebral Fibrocartilage

Fig. 61
Costovertebral Articulations
Anterior View   (Gray)

THE SUBLUXATION OF THE FIRST RIB

A subluxated first rib may be directly involved in three ways in the shoulder, arm and hand syndrome.

1. The first rib is formed, with the grooves and tubercles, to accommodate and transmit such important structures as the subclavian vein, the posterior subclavian artery and the lowest trunk of the brachial plexus. Its tubercles act as attachments and anchorage for the scalenus anterior and the scalenus medius. A subluxation of this rib can cause varying deletrious effects upon these structures.

2. The first rib also acts as the base for the scalene triangle and will become subluxated in the scalene syndrome by the pull of the tense muscles on the rib, thus adding more pressure to the neurovascular bundle. It is essential to correct the subluxated rib in order to give faster and more permanent relief. The first rib also affords the best leverage when correcting the tense muscles.

3. A subluxation of the first rib will narrow the costoclavicular space which causes compression. This will interfere with the neurovascular bundle since these delicate tissues are caught between bones, namely the first rib and the clavicle. It can easily be seen how the subsequent shoulder, arm and hand syndrome may follow when this abnormal condition occurs. All rib subluxations are more to the superior than the posterior because of the transverse process.

LOCATING THE SUBLUXATED FIRST RIB

The subluxated rib can best be palpated at a point approximately four to five inches outward from the spinous process of the first dorsal vertebra, depending upon the size of the patient. If the doctor will palpate both sides simultaneously, the subluxated rib will be quickly detected because it will be higher, more prominent and the muscles in the area will be more tender than on the normal side. In some instances both ribs may be subluxated.

The writer, in his lectures to the chiropractic profession, has many times referred to this misalignment as the chiropractor's subluxation. In our work, the first rib receives a great deal of stress and strain. When an adjustment is given, we rarely bend the elbows and the force is transmitted upward to the region of the first rib. This is comparable to jumping from a four foot height without bending the knees (Fig. 62). The black dot shows the area of tenderness.

THE ADJUSTMENT OF THE FIRST RIB

1. The patient is placed on the adjusting table face down and the doctor stands on the affected side. If it is the right rib, the doctor contacts the rib with his right hand at the base of the index finger (Fig. 63).

2. He then turns the patient's head away from himself and his left hand is placed on the side of the patient's head. The head is then rolled toward the doctor. This relaxes the overlying muscles.

3. While the patient's head is held steady with the left hand, the doctor's right hand is pushed in slowly until all of the slack is taken out of the muscles. The doctor's arm is dropped so that it is parallel with the floor and he stands in such a position that the line of drive will be toward the fourth dorsal. The writer has made it a habit to place his thumb over the patient's shoulder so that the thumb points toward the fourth dorsal (Fig. 63). A short, snappy drive is then given on the first rib while the patient's head is simultaneously rotated toward the doctor's body.

In a number of instances it is advisable to tape the muscles over the rib as shown in Fig. 65. This is simple to do and is a great aid in keeping the rib in place and relaxing the tense muscles.

When the patient is properly positioned and the adjustment correctly executed, it will not harmfully disturb the cervical region, especially not the atlas and axis. In the presence of a scalene syndrome with tense and spastic muscles, this adjustment will have a great beneficial effect upon the involved muscles and the contents of the triangle. The turning of the head will only relax the normal muscles and not the spastic scaleni. However, the adjustment of the first rib will produce a salutary reaction to the involved vertebrae and discs because of their muscular attachment and close relationship to these important structures. This adjustment is not only helpful in correcting the many and varied arm conditions, especially bursitis, but is also very important in relieving shingles affecting the region of the shoulder and arm.

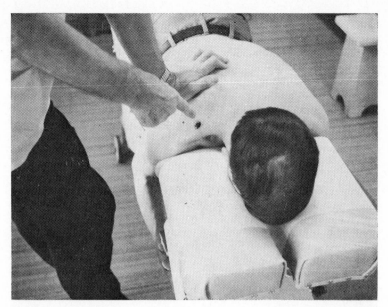

Fig. 62

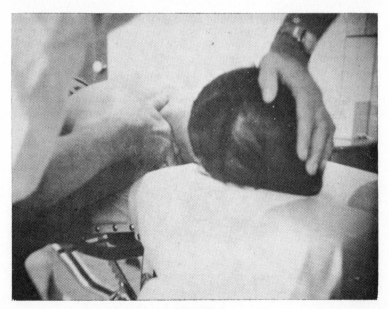

Fig. 63

171

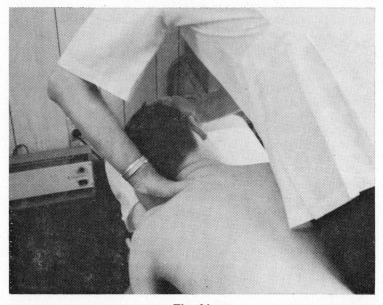

Fig. 64

Alternate move for the first rib. Some doctors may find it more comfortable standing on the opposite side of the rib to be adjusted, as shown above. NOTE: Exactly the same contact is taken at the same distance from the spine as shown in the two foregoing pictures and the thrust is again toward the fourth dorsal vertebra.

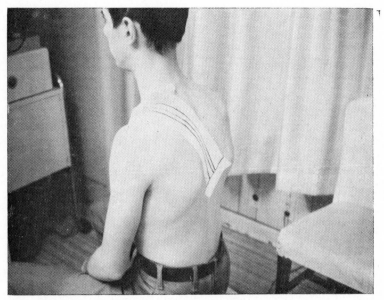

Fig. 65

The taping shown above is used in torticollis, first rib, supraspinatus contraction and, if a wider area is covered, it is an excellent aid in relieving contraction of the rhomboids. The pieces of tape are started in front, about 4 inches below the clavicle, brought up and over the shoulder, then diagonally across the back so that the tape ends on the muscles on the far or opposite side of the spine, and the anchor strips applied as shown. The tension of the tape is from front to back. Folded gauze or cotton may be placed over the area of the supraspinatus to prevent skin irritation. In cases of severe torticollis, the writer tapes the other shoulder in the same manner, forming a "suspender" taping.

173

LOCATING AND ADJUSTING THE SECOND AND THIRD RIBS

The second and third ribs are, in many instances, subluxated along with the first one but they may subluxate alone, without any other rib misalignments. They do not have the close relationship with the neurovascular bundle as does the first rib but are more apt to be the cause of chest pains or intercostal neuralgia.

The point of palpation, which is also the adjustive contact, is on the angle of the rib, close to the tuberosity. This slightly marked angle is approximately two to two and one-half inches from the spinous process of the second or third dorsal vertebra and is about equidistant to the scapular border.

The scapula is used as part of the anchor point and shield for the thrust given by the adjustive hand. In fact, as much of the hand as possible is placed upon the scapula when making the contact point. About two-thirds of the hand is on the scapula and only a small portion contacts the rib angle. The writer, in using these rib adjustments in all the years of practice, has never injured a rib, much less cracked one, because the scapula dissipates much of the force of the thrust.

If it is the patient's left second or third rib that is to be adjusted, the doctor stands on the left side of the adjusting table with the patient in the face down position. Approximately two-thirds of the left hand is placed on the patient's right scapula with the pisiform in contact with the rib angle. Then the patient's head is turned toward the doctor and he then places his left hand on the side of the patient's head (Fig. 67). With moderate pressure on the scapula, the doctor then pushes the patient's head away from himself in order to take the slack from the muscles. With the pisiform on the contact point, the patient's head is pushed away from the doctor while he simultaneously gives a short, fast thrust upon the scapula. The doctor stands in such a position that the line of drive is not straight downward but rather down and at the same time to the inferior. When the adjustment is made, the scapula will give just enough and the rib will be adjusted by the pisiform contact. The movement will be felt and it is almost always audible.

This adjustment is not at all painful and it is safe because the contact is not taken on the rib alone. To adjust the right second or third ribs, reverse all contacts.

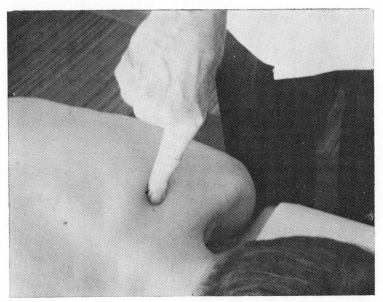
Fig. 66
Locating third rib

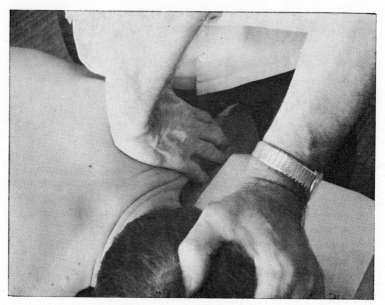

Fig. 67
Showing pisiform contact

MOVE TWO—ALTERNATE METHOD

Many doctors are either extremely right or left handed, so it may be easier, in either of these situations, to use this alternate method (Fig. 68).

Step 1. The patient lies face down on the adjusting table. If it is the left rib, the doctor stands on the right side of the table, placing his right hand on the patient's scapula with about two-thirds of the pisiform side of the hand in contact with it. The base of the first metacarpus is placed upon the rib to be adjusted (Fig. 68).

Step 2. The doctor's left hand is placed upon the opposite scapula to steady the patient when the thrust is given. The doctor then positions himself so that the line of drive on the scapula and rib will be downward and to the inferior. He then gives a short, snappy thrust. This will usually give a satisfactory correction and may be more comfortable to the patient since this area of the hand is softer than when the pisiform contact is used. Reverse all contacts when adjusting the right second rib by this method.

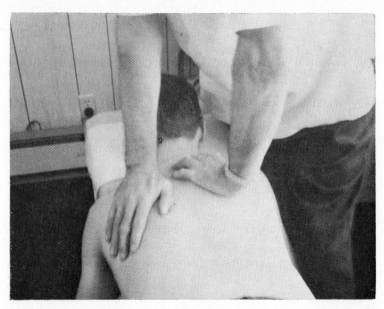

Fig. 68

Alternate move for the second or third ribs. First metacarpal contact shown.

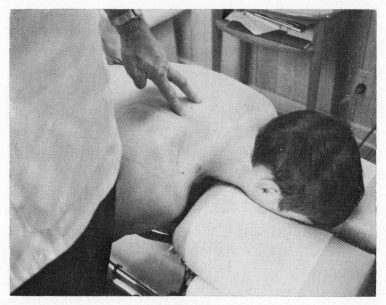

Fig. 69

The above picture shows the distance of the scapula from the spine, the index finger locating the contact point for the adjustment of the fourth or fifth ribs which should be just off the edge of the scapula. Either the pisiform contact shown in Fig. 70 or the first metacarpal contact shown in Fig. 71 may be used.

178

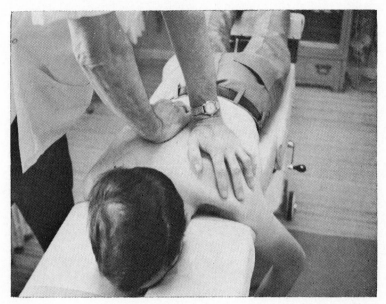

Fig. 70
Pisiform contact

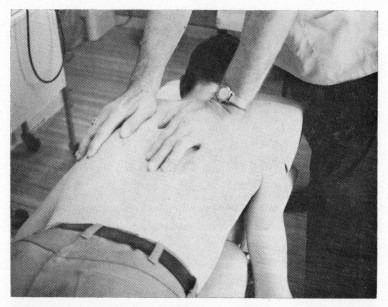

Fig. 71

Showing the first metacarpal contact. As long as contact can be maintained with the scapula, this method could be used as low as the eighth or ninth ribs. When contacting the last two mentioned, it may be advantageous to have the patient, if possible, place his forearm on his back at the waistline. This will usually draw the scapula inward.

In some rare cases, such as in a violent accident, a rib or ribs may be subluxated to the inferior. If the doctor's palpation indicates this possibility, x-ray films should be made of the area and, if confirmed, the ribs should be adjusted from the inferior. The move shown above in Fig. 71 could be used in reverse.

SUBLUXATIONS OF THE STERNOCOSTAL ARTICULATIONS

Subluxations in these articulations are rather uncommon but can occur from a fall or violent accident. By palpation, the misalignments will be noted and pain elicited. There will also be pain in the intercostal spaces on the lateral, anterior chest wall.

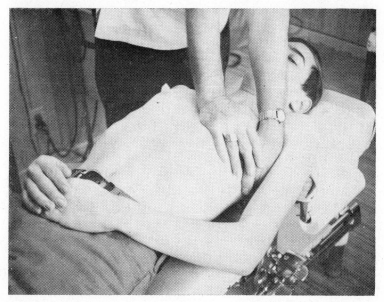

Fig. 72

The above picture shows the left side being adjusted. The doctor's left hand contacts the scapula and raises the patient's shoulder slightly upward. While holding it in this somewhat elevated position, his right hand gives a short, light, downward thrust.

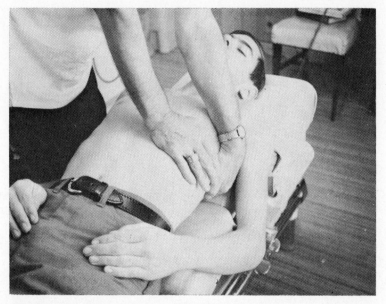

Fig. 73

To adjust the lower true ribs, the lower rib cage is contacted and raised slightly while the right hand gives a short, light thrust.

Both of these moves produce great leverage and for that reason the doctor must be sure that the thrust given is both light and short.

The scapula can certainly be called "the home base from which seventeen muscles operate" (Fig. 74). It also gives reception to the head of the humerus into which these muscles are inserted. Any one, or any group of these muscles, when in a state of contraction, may cause a marked effect upon the arm from a sensory, vascular or motor standpoint. A number of these muscles have the neuro-vascular bundle running directly underneath them which places the bundle in close proximity to bone. In other words, these important nerves, arteries and veins run through a channel composed of muscle and bone, and therefore the effect of a contracted muscle or muscle group upon these important structures can easily be visualized. A good example is the coracoid process and a shortened pectoralis minor (Fig. 3).

Another important group of muscles that frequently become contracted are those at the posterior portion of the shoulder, namely, the triceps, the teres major and minor. Though the latissimus dorsi is attached to the scapula only by way of union with the teres major in a small area at its lower border, it must be reckoned with not only because of its great power, but also because it lies in close proximity to the above mentioned three muscles and because it is attached to the humerus (Fig. 80).

The space formed by this muscular arrangement is known as the quadrangular space. It is roofed above by the inferior portion of the glenoid, the neck of the scapula, the head of the humerus and the capsule. Constriction of one of these muscles, of two or three or of the entire group, may cause pressure on the vessels and the circumflex nerve which pass close to the bony roof above, along with the radial and triceps nerves (Fig. 81). Any of these muscles, when contracted, should be manipulated and adjusted specifically as shown on pages 188, 189, 190, 191 and 192.

The writer has found that in many cases, one scapula is more moveable than the other and some appear to be practically adhesed to the posterior chest wall. In dealing with these cases, the doctor will find that the affected arm is always on the side of the fixed scapula, and results will not be forthcoming to the patient until the scapula is freed from the contracted muscles. It is not at all unusual to have patients present themselves with bilateral involvement and these persons are truly in misery.

The most unusual case of the latter—bilateral involvement—that has ever come to the writer's attention was that of a young

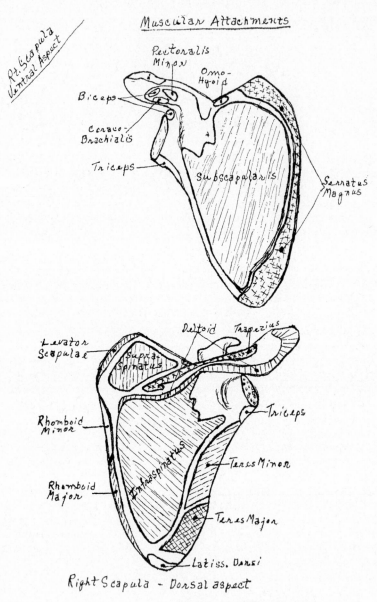

Rt. Scapula
Ventral Aspect

Pectoralis
Minor

Omo-
Hyoid

Biceps

Coraco-
Brachialis

Triceps

Subscapularis

Serratus
Magnus

Levator
Scapulae

Deltoid

Trapezius

Supra-
Spinatus

Triceps

Rhomboid
Minor

Infraspinatus

Teres Minor

Rhomboid
Major

Teres Major

Latiss. Dorsi

Right Scapula – Dorsal aspect

Fig. 74

woman who came to the office about two years ago. She was then 21 years old, three years married and was a tiny person of 100 pounds. She kept up a small house and worked part time as a secretary. Her complaint was pain—pain all over but the worst of it was situated from between the shoulders to the back of the neck and her arms. She had frequent severe headaches and the pains in her worst areas ranged from aching to gnawing to throbbing. Her arms fell asleep and occasionally would swell and she said she was completely exhausted at all times to the extent that on many days she could not do her housework.

She had sought medical help and was given varying diagnoses ranging from incipient arthritis to it being a psychosomatic problem. At that point she turned to chiropractic and had two adjustments a week for a little over two years. Though she had gone to a doctor who is known to be very competent, her problem remained. At that point she came to our office.

She was given a complete physical examination with negative results. The x-ray films showed no bony pathology; they showed the usual spinal misalignments that are to be expected with her case history. However, both first ribs were extremely high, the right being more so than the left. The head of the right humerus was drawn posteriorly, the left one less so, and there was slight disc compression in the mid-dorsal area. Upon examination, her scapulae were found to be nearly completely adhesed and she could barely produce movement when asked to adduct them. She could not, without considerable discomfort, put her hands behind her back at the waistline. Head movements were somewhat restricted.

Knowing that the spinal adjustments that this young woman had received before she came in were as good as those that we could give, it was obvious that a different approach was necessary in an effort to give her relief. Therefore, along with the spinal adjustments, muscle adjustments were used, the first ribs were adjusted along with correction of the humeral misalignments.

All of the corrective procedures used are shown in Figs. 63 and 75 to 86 inclusive. In a severe case of fixation, such as this one, it is only reasonable to expect some discomfort during the correction and the patient must have the situation explained to him. This was done in her case and the first muscle adjustments were done easily. After a few office calls she said, "I feel different. Go ahead and work. If I can't stand it, I'll tell you." She never made a complaint, but a few times she did give a big sigh.

This patient was adjusted twice a week for three months, then once a week for five and a half months at which time she appeared to be completely pain free. Since that time she has appeared at the office every month saying, "I don't ever want to hurt again like I did; that is why I'm here."

The cause of her condition? There was no history of accident of any kind. Neither she, her mother or sister could think of anything, yet she had been in this pain since the age of fourteen. The cause WAS finally located, and it was this: She grew up on a farm in a family of girls. Outside help was desperately needed and in the absence of boys, the girls were called upon. Therefore she was carrying large pails of feed and water from the time that she could possibly do so until her marriage at 18, and this daily overlifting, even though no real accident ever occurred, laid the groundwork for the muscle contractions that were never allowed to recede because of the constant aggravation. She was, in effect, making her "Volkswagon sized" body do the work of an International truck. She was therefore instructed in the proper methods of carrying or lifting loads that were suitable to her size and told never again to attempt overloads.

The muscles that are most generally involved, one or more at a time, and those that can be specifically adjusted, are the following: the pectoralis minor, infraspinatus, supraspinatus, teres major, teres minor, the levator scapulae, rhomboid major, rhomboid minor, short head of the biceps, coracobrachialis, the trapezius and latissimus dorsi. The remainder of the muscles attached to the scapula are adjusted indirectly (Figs. 75 to 100 inclusive).

THE QUADRANGLE

The quadrilateral space and muscles in the immediate area are very important in the correction of nearly all shoulder lesions. This space is bounded above by the neck of the scapula, the inferior aspect of the glenoid, the inferior glenoid tuberosity, the capsule and the humeral head. The lower boundary is formed by the criss-crossing of the long head of the triceps and the teres major. The teres minor and the upper part of the latissimus dorsi are also closely associated with this area. This space contains the circumflex nerve, artery and vein, the radial nerve and branches of the triceps. The muscles of this region, when tense or injured, may constrict this space and squeeze these important nerves and vessels against the long boundary above (Fig. 81).

The adjustive moves used in manipulating and relaxing these

muscles are shown in Figs. 75 through 79. The one shown in Fig. 77 also has a marked effect in separating the head of the humerus from its adhesed association with the glenoid. This move should be used gently at first, then gradually increased to the patient's tolerance and the arm should never be roughly forced or twisted. It must be remembered that the treatment is for the purpose of correcting the involved subluxations, stretching and loosening the adhesions, relaxing the tense muscles and improving their power so that increased movement may be obtained.

In order to more easily remember the five salient points that must be kept in mind when treating this kind of shoulder condition, they can be summarized as follows: THE FROZEN SHOULDER QUINTUPLETS are the adjustment of the SPINE, RIBS and MUSCLES, EXERCISES and TIME. Because the frozen shoulder is a resulting and rarely a primary condition, the underlying causes must be thoroughly sought out and patiently treated. Without a doubt, this type of situation is the most difficult of shoulder cases.

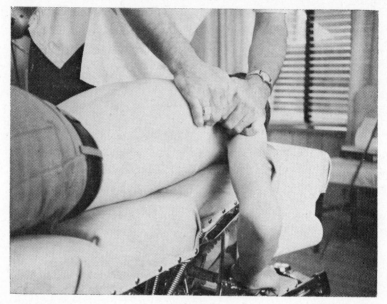

Fig. 75

The above photograph and the following four show the methods of adjusting and manipulating the quadrangular space. This is a most important area when caring for the stubborn arm and shoulder conditions, and manipulation will have a beneficial effect in two ways, namely, relief of pain and increased moveability of the arm. The above photograph shows the position of the patient, the doctor and the doctor's hands and fingers. The fingertips will be on the area of tenderness. From this contact, the fingers should enforce an upward pressure, or lifting of the muscles. Begin gently and increase to the patient's tolerance.

The anatomical diagrams relating to this adjustment are found on pages 193 and 194.

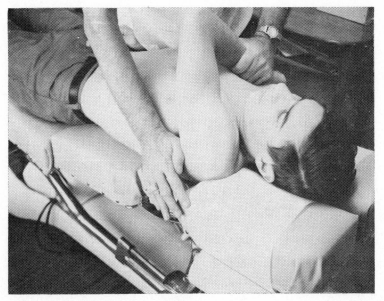

Fig. 76

This picture shows the second step. The patient is placed as shown and the doctor stands on the opposite side of the affected muscles and grasps the patient's affected arm above the wrist and places it across his chest. Then the doctor places his other hand in the quadrangular space and uses gentle downward pressure while simultaneously pulling the arm toward himself.

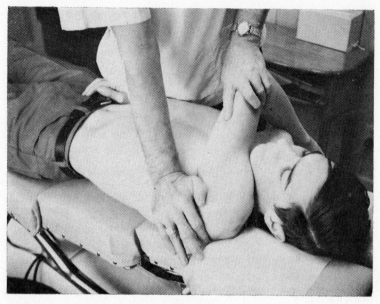

Fig. 77

This picture shows a more forceful method and is not usually used in the first treatment if the patient is in great pain. Note that the doctor's hand is now just above the patient's elbow and this produces a great deal of leverage. The hand on the muscle uses a firm downward pressure while the other hand simultaneously pushes the patient's elbow to the opposite side of his body. Because of the great leverage involved, the move should be begun gently and then increased to the patient's tolerance. When this area is involved, four or five adjustments will show marked improvement; however, not all arm complaints will exhibit tenderness in this specific area.

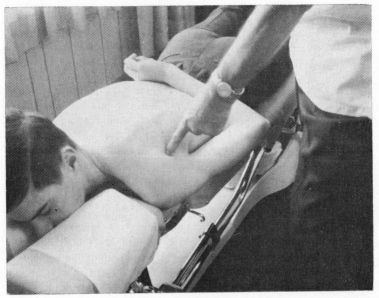

Fig. 78

The above photograph shows the point of posterior tenderness which is located just at the edge of the posterior portion of the deltoid. Note the position of the patient's arm.

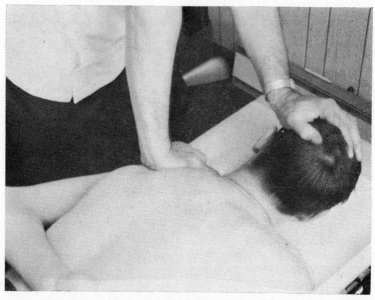

Fig. 79

With the patient in position as shown, the doctor takes a pisiform contact over the point of tenderness. With his other hand he steadies the patient's head in a position slightly away from the affected side. Then a fast, short drive is given downward and to the inferior.

A tense deltoid can also be adjusted in the manner above EXCEPT the contact point is about an inch **upward** from the one shown. CAUTION: This is a soft tissue contact, therefore it is extremely important that the doctor NEVER take the contact too high, in which case it would be over the posterior head of the humerus and could produce an anterior humeral subluxation.

Of all the stubborn shoulder cases that have come into the writer's office, the most dramatic results have been obtained with the above outlined method.

192

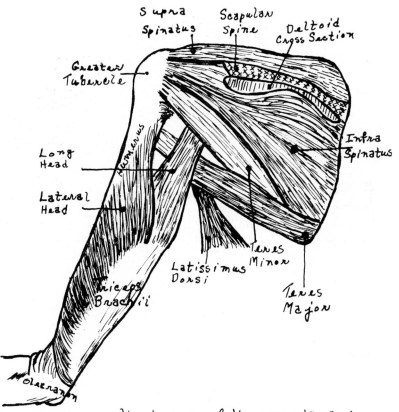

Supra Spinatus   Scapular Spine   Deltoid Cross Section

Greater Tubercle

Humerus

Long Head

Lateral Head

Infra Spinatus

Triceps Brachii

Latissimus Dorsi

Teres Minor

Teres Major

Olecranon

Muscles on the dorsum of the scapula and the Triceps Brachii   (Gray)

Fig. 80

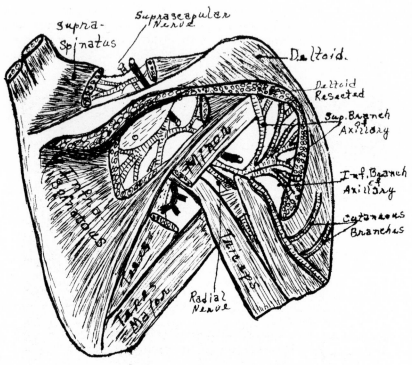

Fig. 81
Suprascapular and Axillary Nerves
Right Side From Behind   (Gray)

194

THE ADJUSTMENT AND MANIPULATION OF THE RHOMBOIDS

The two rhomboids are important muscles in the maintenance of posture and when in a state of contraction, the subject cannot raise the arm above shoulder level. These muscles are mostly covered by the trapezius except at the lower border of the scapula. For that reason the trapezius is also manipulated when executing this correction.

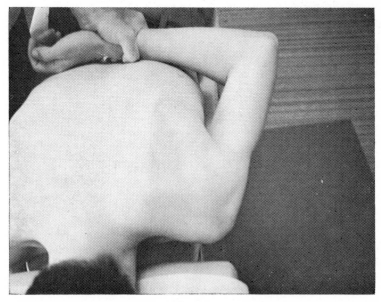

Fig. 82

1. The above photograph shows the correct positioning of the patient's arm for this adjustment. It can be seen that the scapula is somewhat raised, which allows for better contact. Note the amount of space between the angle of the elbow and the body. This space should NOT be decreased, both for the comfort of the patient and to avoid strain on the shoulder joint.

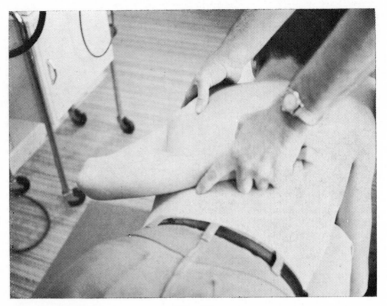

Fig. 83

2. This picture shows the border of the scapula with the doctor's thumb in the approximate center of the two muscles. Without pulling on the arm, but holding it firmly on the back, the doctor prods the entire length of the medial scapular border with his thumb in order to determine tension and tenderness. In cases of extreme tenderness, the thumb may be used to manipulate the muscles, working up and down the scapular border a number of times with a kneading, pushing pressure.

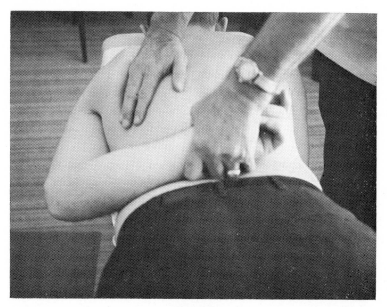

Fig. 84

The above picture shows the manipulation of the muscles with the side of the hand, pushing the scapula outward and upward from the posterior chest wall while holding the bent arm firmly but WITHOUT PULLING on it. At first, the doctor may find it almost impossible to get even the lateral side of the little finger under the edge of the scapula but after four or five treatments, the small and ring fingers will easily slide under it, without any discomfort to the patient.

These cases will complain of pain between the shoulders, difficulty in raising the arms and, very often, also of chest pains. A few patients will not be able to get their arm in the position shown, in which case the rhomboids and adjacent muscles must be adjusted with the arms in the usual forward position until they are loose enough to allow the arm to be placed on the back.

197

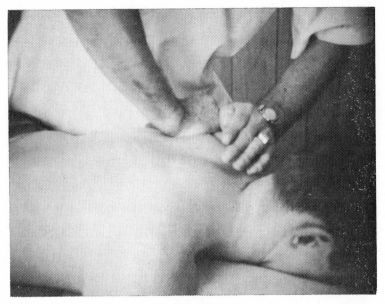

Fig. 85

The above picture and the following one show methods of loosening all muscles attached to the scapula, and is especially useful in those cases where the patient cannot bring his arm to the back as shown in the preceding photographs. In this picture the doctor's left hand is on the superior border of the scapula pushing medialward and the right hand on the medial-inferior scapular border pushing laterally. This gives a stretching effect to the muscles. This move should be done repeatedly, each time giving a firm stretch.

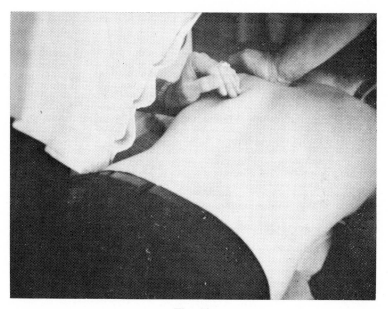

Fig. 86

The move pictured above is particularly effective in relieving tension in the serratus anterior muscle and the tendon of the subscapularis. The doctor's right hand is placed at the superior-medial scapular border and pushes laterally while the left hand is placed at the lateral-inferior scapular border and pushes medially. In both of these photographs, reverse the contact positions for the right side of the patient's body.

THE CORACOID PROCESS AND THE PECTORALIS MINOR

The coracoid process is a thumb-like projection from the neck of the scapula and important structures are attached to it. The great vessels run beneath it and it is also an important landmark. It is palpated just below the lateral end of the clavicle, projecting slightly outward underneath the medial border of the deltoid muscle. Attached to the tip and extending toward the chest wall is the pectoralis minor. This muscle is small and thick, arising from the third, fourth and fifth ribs.

The great vessels and nerves of the arm pass beneath the pectoralis minor on their course to the arm and hand. By pressing just below the coracoid process, the pulsating of the artery may be felt. It is possible for pathological processes to compress the neurovascular bundle in this area. The subclavian artery and vein, accompanied by three fibers of the brachial plexus come out from under the clavicle. They are enveloped in a sleeve from the clavopectoral fascia and continue down the cervico-axillary canal. Sometimes this edge is thickened and contains cartilage. Tightening or thickening of this structure may compress the neurovascular bundle.

The cervico-axillary canal is roofed by the clavicle, subclavian fascia and the pectoralis minor. The fascial connection may, through certain conditions, conduct traction force, compressing the neurovascular bundle in extreme extension and lateral rotation. Certain movements, such as abduction, external rotation and extension, can compress the neurovascular bundle against the head of the humerus. This is the position sometimes assumed in sleep and is a frequent cause of radiating discomfort.

Most often the musculofascial tension can be relieved by using the adjustive methods described on page 202 (Fig. 88). Two other important muscles are also attached to the coracoid process, namely, the coraco-brachialis and the short head of the biceps brachii. Tension and tenderness in them can be detected by palpation and, when present, should also be adjusted as shown in Figs. 88 and 89.

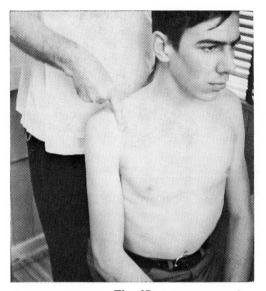

Fig. 87

This photograph shows the location of the insertion of the pectoralis minor at the coracoid, which will be tender when the muscle is involved. With the finger in the position shown, glide it slightly downward and medialward about an inch. That will be the point of tenderness when there is involvement of the pectoralis minor.

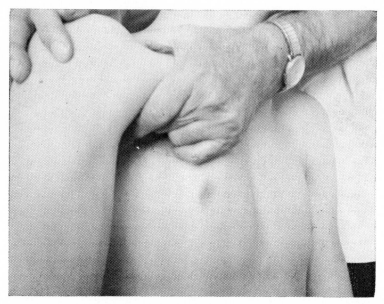

Fig. 88

This photograph shows the contact for the adjustment of the pectoralis minor with the doctor standing opposite the affected side. With the hand in position, the fingers are slowly worked upward until muscle resistance is felt. At that point, the fingers are worked upward again, but at the same time, also to the posterior. This procedure may have to be repeated two or three times before it is possible to reach the deep area to be adjusted. When the fingers cannot travel any farther, the doctor gives a short, swift move obliquely **outward** toward his own body. Caution: This move should never be given in a straight upward thrust since it could be possible to injure the neurovascular bundle by pushing it against the hard, bony coracoid process. See Figs. 3, 90, 91 for the anatomical structures involved.

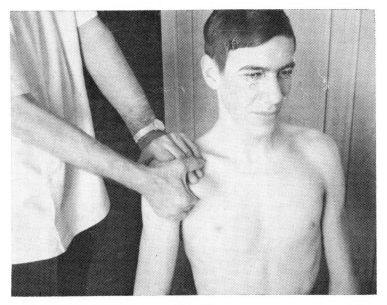

Fig. 89

The adjustment of the short head of the biceps and coracobrachialis. When these muscles are involved, tenderness will be found at or near the coracoid process, their site of attachment. The adjustment to relieve this tension is somewhat similar to that used on the pectoralis minor, Fig. 88. However, the doctor stands ON the affected side and the short, fast pull is made TOWARD his own body. See Figs. 3 and 91 for the anatomy involved.

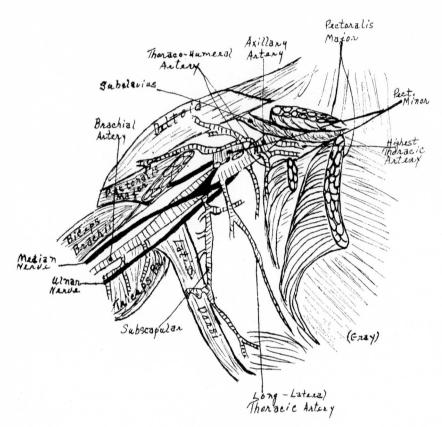

Fig. 90
The Axillary Artery and
its branches (Gray)

204

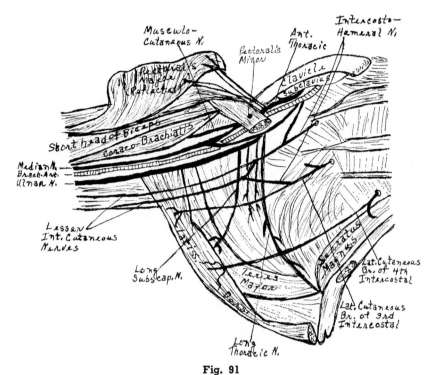

Fig. 91

Right Brachial Plexus Viewed From Below and in Front.
Pectoralis Major and Minor Largely Removed
and Their Attachments Reflected.   (Gray)

ADJUSTMENT OF THE SUPRASPINATUS

The supraspinatus occupies the whole of the supraspinatus fossa and it fixes the head of the humerus in its movement in the glenoid cavity. It is a part of the rotor cuff. The anatomical relationships are shown in schematic drawings on pages 193 and 194.

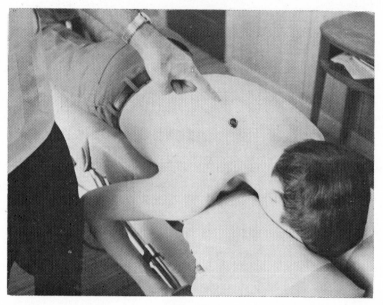

Fig. 92

The whole of the muscle is tender when it is in a state of contraction but the above located area is the point of greatest discomfort.

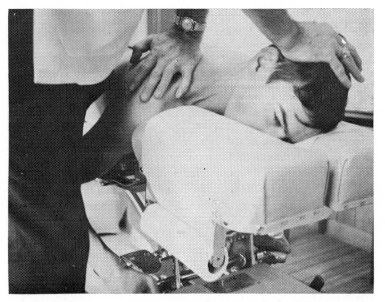

Fig. 93

A pisiform contact is taken over the superior margin of the supraspinatus. The doctor's other hand turns the patient's head slightly away from the affected side and he stands as far headward of the patient as possible while still being able to hold firm contact.

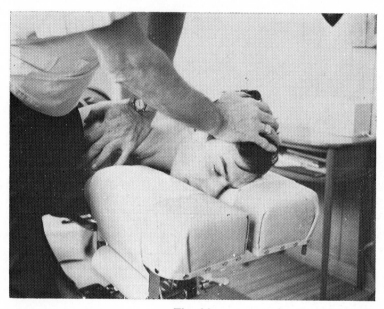

Fig. 94

The thrust is given downward and inferiorly while simultaneously holding firm pressure on the head.

THE ADJUSTMENT OF THE INFRASPINATUS

The infraspinatus occupies the chief part of the infraspinatus fossa and also aids in the formation of the rotor cuff. The schematic drawings of the anatomical relationships of this area are shown on pages 193 and 194.

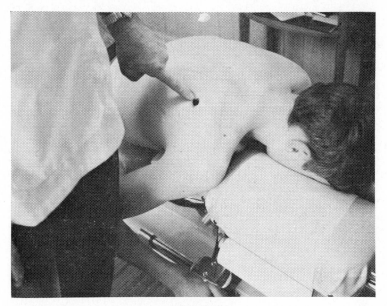

Fig. 95

In the above photograph, the darkened area being pointed out is the usual trigger point in the infraspinatus syndrome. Pressure on this area or rolling of the muscle with the finger produces, and/or intensifies the pain in this already painful syndrome. Therefore, the object is to work close to and around it, but never directly on it.

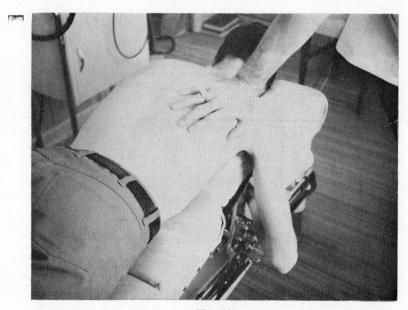

Fig. 96

This picture shows the contact and direction of drive. The heel of the doctor's hand is placed on the superior part of the infraspinatus just below the supraspinatus fossa, making sure to be just off the trigger point.

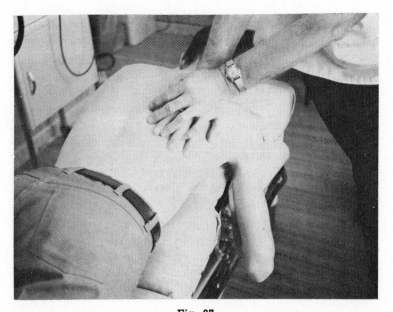

Fig. 97

Here the completed contact is shown. The doctor then gives a short, fast thrust downward and medially toward the spine.

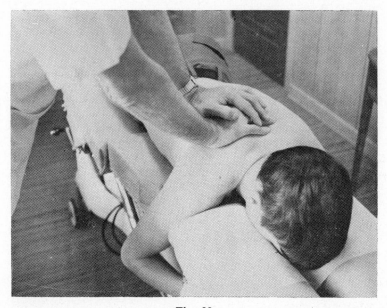

Fig. 98

Next, the muscle is adjusted from the lateral aspect as shown above. The heel of the doctor's one hand contacts the lateral border of the infraspinatus, being sure not to be directly on the trigger point. His other hand is placed over the first one in the same manner as shown in Fig. 97. He then gives three or four thrusts in quick succession, the line of drive being directly toward the spine.

This is a very important correction in a great number of shoulder cases because of the power of the muscle, its action on the humerus and its relation to the rotor cuff. It is not a painful move unless the contact is made on the trigger point.

THE ADJUSTMENT OF THE LEVATOR SCAPULAE

This is a very important muscle to adjust in all cases of arm pain. It is also important because of its connection with the cervical region, originating from the transverse processes of the five upper cervical vertebrae.

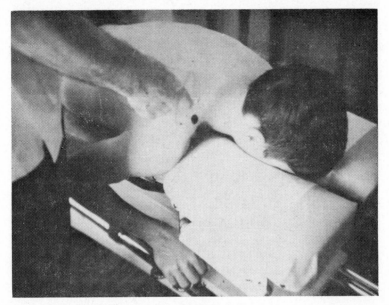

Fig. 99

This picture shows the location of the tender area at the upper margin of the scapula. It lies just under the trapezius, which may also evidence tenderness.

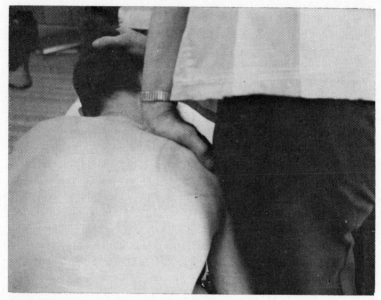

Fig. 100

The above photograph shows the contact over the tender area. The doctor's other hand is placed on the patient's head, pushing it slightly away. The thrust is given quickly downward and to the inferior while at the same time holding the head steady.

Chapter X
DISORDERS OF THE ELBOW, WRIST AND HAND

DISORDERS OF THE ELBOW

There are two types of lesions in elbow disorders, namely the extra-articular and intra-articular. The term "tennis elbow" appears to be a common one for all disabilities of the elbow joint, much as the term "lumbago" is used to cover most lower back disorders.

THE EXTRA-ARTICULAR LESION:

The commonest cause of pain in the elbow usually is a lesion of some sort affecting the extensor muscles of the forearm close to their origins on the lateral side of the elbow and which is generally caused by a minor strain or overuse of the arm. It is noteable that few of the muscle fibers are inserted directly into the bone, but rather, most arise from the ligaments, fascia and intermuscular septa which are relatively mobile.

It is this situation that makes it difficult to coordinate the contraction of the individual fibers, for example, when the hand is in the act of gripping firmly while at the same time, the elbow is extended or the forearm is in the act of rotation. Investigators have failed to explain the real nature of the lesion, which could be one of a number of things, such as a sprain or strain, inflammation of the intermuscular fibrous tissue or a disturbance of local metabolism. In the absence of a defined localized cause, the onset has been attributed to cervical spondylosis. However, it would appear necessary to also look to the spine for cervical subluxations, upper dorsal misalignments, scalene syndrome involvement and subluxations of the first rib.

SYMPTOMS. There is a history of pain, usually of a gradual onset, which the patient may attribute to tennis, throwing a baseball or an occupation that involved much use of the forearm, such as the use of a screwdriver by a woodworking hobbyist who is unaccustomed to the work. The pain may not be noticed at the time the work is being done but becomes apparent soon afterward, perhaps the following day. At times the onset is abrupt and is associated readily with a certain strain. The pain is relieved by rest but returns when the arm is again used. Excessive use may cause a widespread aching in the muscles of the forearm, especially when the occupation or sport requires the tight gripping of an object along with rotation of the arm.

In such instances the area of acute tenderness can be localized accurately. The usual site is over and just in front of the collateral ligament (Figs. 8 and 101). During the acute stage there is, at times, diffuse tenderness over the extensor muscles and the triceps brachii is the main great extensor of the forearm (Fig. 80). There is normal or nearly normal range of active and passive movements; however, pain is caused by extension of the elbow and is usually increased by pronating the affected arm and flexing the wrist while the elbow is extended. Only occasionally is the pain increased by supinating the forearm and extending the wrist. In chronic lesions the pain may spread over the back of the forearm. In those cases the fascia has become thick and inflamed and x-rays are generally negative.

TREATMENT. Lesions of this type do not respond to treatment as readily as do most minor injuries and sprains. Most cases are very stubborn. Even when nearly healed, the symptoms return when the arm is used too vigorously so it follows that there should be complete freedom from pain and tenderness before the patient can return to a strenuous occupation. The earlier the patient begins treatment the better the prognosis and the quicker the cure.

The first step in case management is to tape the area in the manner outlined in Figs. 103 and 104. If the pain area has spread over the entire forearm and extends to the wrist, place an old nylon stocking over the forearm and apply the tape over the whole pain area. Leave it in place for from several days to a week. It is essential that the extensor muscles have a complete rest for ten to twelve days. The use of a sling is advisable in most instances. The writer has found that a knitted ankle support is very useful to give support after the tape is removed, placing it so that the olecranon process of the elbow goes through the heel opening. Most people do not seek help soon enough, dismissing the condition as trivial. They will even doubt the advice on the necessity of a sling. A small bursa lying deep in the extensor muscles may, on occasion, also be involved and cause much pain.

If the patient has a history of a fall, an occupation or sport where the arm has been put under great strain, the head of the radius may be subluxated. Palpation will elicit tenderness and, when compared with the normal arm, fullness will be noted. If present, the misalignment should be corrected as shown in Fig. 102.

216

SUBLUXATION OF THE RADIUS

The adjustment of radial subluxations has been found to be very helpful in cases of numb or "sleeping" fingers. The writer has found that many persons who use a typewriter request this move once they have had it, because of the relief that it brings. He has also found that, in practically all cases of a sprained wrist, the radius is subluxated. This was forcefully brought to his attention when a young girl, who had fallen at the bus depot, was brought to his office with a severely sprained wrist. Cold applications were used and a strong taping was applied. One week later, the girl's sister called and said that the wrist "didn't look right" and that a bone was "sticking up" at the side of the wrist. Upon examination it was found that the distal end of the ulna was much higher than that of the normal wrist. There was no tenderness on or around the olecranon process, however, the radius, at the site of its head, was extremely tender and appeared fuller when compared with the normal one.

The radius was adjusted as shown in Fig. 102 and much to his surprise, the end of the ulna appeared to be in normal position. Knowing that he had not adjusted the ulna, it took several hours of thinking in order to ascertain how the correction was brought about and how it was possible since the lower extremity of the radius articulates with the ulna, navicular and lunate. The adjustment corrected the misalignment of these bones, however, it was the radius that was out of position, and, when corrected, the wrist again had a normal appearance and was free of discomfort. The writer's explanation of this is that the radius was lower than the ulna and the correction normalized and leveled it.

THE ADJUSTMENT OF THE RADIAL HEAD

To locate the exact area of tenderness, the doctor grasps the patient's affected arm just above the wrist and rotates it inward. The area pointed out in Fig. 101 will evidence fullness and palpation will elicit tenderness. It should also be remembered that when there is a misalignment between the radius and ulna, there is also a subluxation between the radial head and distal end of the humerus.

To adjust the radial head as shown in Fig. 102, the doctor grasps the forearm JUST above the wrist and, with the arm fully extended, turns it inward until the olecranon process is pointed almost directly upward. Then with the other hand, the doctor takes

217

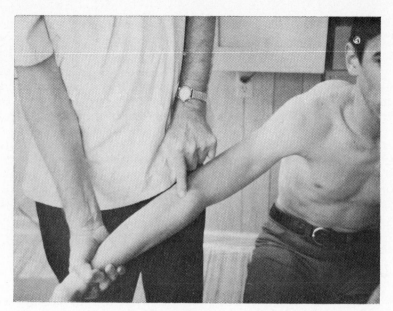

Fig. 101

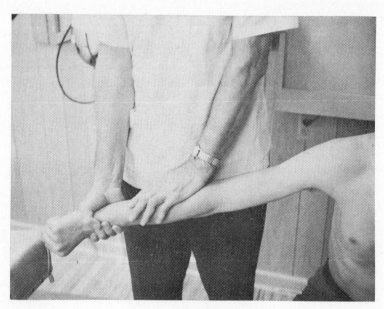

Fig. 102

a pisiform contact on the radius as shown and pushes the joint slightly forward or downward to remove muscular slack. At this point he simultaneously places a very firm pressure on the distal end of the forearm and gives a short, fast thrust to the radial head.

It is not at all unusual for the radius to be subluxated at both ends and for that reason, the firm pressure on its distal end will aid that end in realignment. At times, this move will produce a shock-like pain for just a second, and because of this, it should be done very quickly. It is a very beneficial adjustment that will give relief in a wide array of arm difficulties.

BURSITIS OF THE ELBOW JOINT

This condition is most often caused by a bump on the posterior part of the elbow, though it may also appear after some unusual work in which pressure is brought to bear upon this portion of the elbow. It is similar to housemaid's knee or bursitis of the knee. Usually it is not too painful a situation and a taping, such as shown in Figs. 103 and 104, brings prompt relief. The writer has also found that an elastic ankle support, worn with the heel opening on the inside of the elbow, is very helpful. By wearing the opening to the inside of the joint, it allows complete closure over the olecranon process which produces beneficial pressure. When tape is applied, the arm must be in the extended position.

EXTERNAL EPICONDYLITIS AND TENDINITIS OF THE ELBOW

This is a situation in which the lateral epicondyle is tender on pressure, along with the tendons of the biceps and brachialis. They will feel raised and can easily be rolled under the fingers. These symptoms may also be associated with numbness and tingling of the fingers. The pain is aggravated by grasping an object with all fingertips and exerting a squeezing pressure. This will cause pain in the region of the elbow and the extensors below it. In many cases the tendons are so contracted that the patient cannot fully extend the arm.

The difficulty is usually caused by doing a job to which the individual is unaccustomed. Many of these cases appear during harvest time when shoveling of grain is required or during the haying season when heavy bales must be thrown into place, or in any industrial occupations where the forearm is strained. Usually the triceps tendon is also involved since the triceps is the great extensor of the arm and is a direct antagonist of the biceps brachii and the brachialis (Fig. 80).

219

TAPING FOR BURSITIS OF THE ELBOW

This taping must be applied with the elbow straight for the reason that when the arm is flexed it will create pressure on the accumulated fluid and aid lymphatic drainage. Four strips of tape are criss-crossed over the posterior part of the elbow as shown in Fig. 103. About ten strips are placed over the criss-crossed pieces as shown (Fig. 104). On the inside of the elbow, the ends of the applied tape should be an inch or two apart. To anchor, take three pieces of tape, three inches long, and LAY them across the open area, two below the joint and one above. The anchor strips should not have any pull or pressure applied to them, since they simply are to hold the ends of the previously applied tape in place. The width of the tape used is inch and a half.

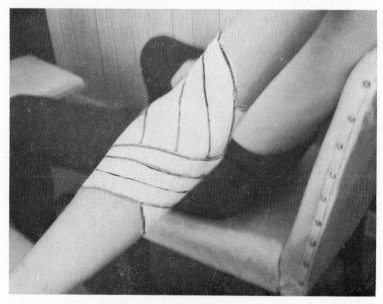

Fig. 103
First Taping — Posterior Aspect

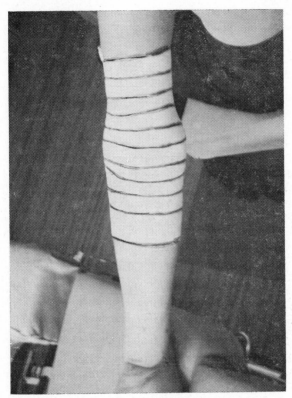

Fig. 104
Second Taping — Posterior Aspect

CASE MANAGEMENT OF EXTERNAL EPICONDYLITIS
AND TENDINITIS

When the patient presents himself at the office, it is advisable to apply heat, by way of a heat lamp or hot packs, and then to gently manipulate the tendons from side to side. In most instances, the doctor will find subluxations either in the cervical area, the upper dorsal region or in the area of the first rib. When any of these areas present misalignments, they should be corrected. Then the elbow should have a strong taping applied to the front and sides while it is in a partially flexed position (Fig. 105). Thereafter, rest for from three to five days is essential.

When the patient returns for his second appointment the same procedure should be followed, except that an ankle support may be placed on the elbow with the heel opening over the olecranon. The patient, after this office visit, should be advised to stretch the tendons by placing the hand over the top of a door and pulling downward with a part of his weight—up to his tolerance (Fig. 141). This has a beneficial effect upon the tendons and the arm will soon straighten. In most cases, it is not advisable to use adjustments while in the acute stage because of the extreme tendon contraction. However, later the radius should be checked for misalignment and adjusted if necessary.

INTERARTICULAR ELBOW DISORDERS

This type of disorder is not uncommon and is caused by a sport or occupation where the elbow articulation is put to great strain and overuse. Authorities believe that, in all probability, a small portion of the synovial membrane is nipped between the articular surfaces of the radius and humerus in the same way that tissues may be nipped between the bones of the knee. Unless the fringe of the synovial membrane is released within a short period of time, it may become edematous and slough and then a raw, tender spot is the result which, in turn, will adhere to another part of the synovial membrane, thereby forming an adhesion.

TAPING FOR TENDINITIS OF THE ELBOW

When applying a taping for this condition, the arm MUST be flexed to a degree slightly less than a right angle and the tape is applied to the inside of the joint. The first layer is again applied in a criss-cross manner using three or four strips on each side (Fig. 105). In Fig. 106 the strips that run across the first taping are shown. It will take about ten or twelve and they are applied with firm pressure against the arm. Again, the arm is not encircled. The

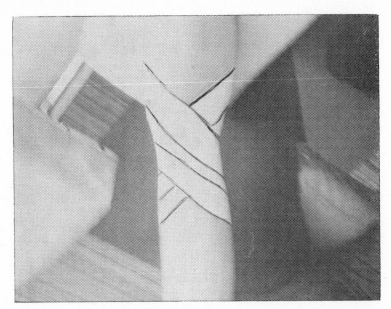

Fig. 105

First Taping — Anterior Aspect

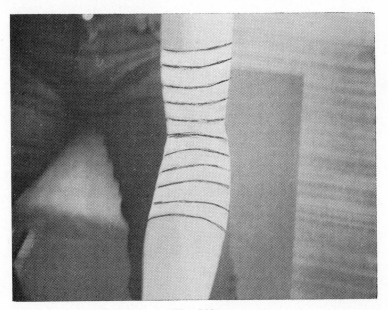

Fig. 106

Second Taping — Anterior Aspect

tape ends on the back of the articulation should be about one to two inches apart. Anchor them with three three-inch long strips— two below the elbow and one above—and apply them without any pressure or pull.

SYMPTOMS: There will be a history of pain of sudden occurrence during the course of action, either athletic or occupational, when the arm is used extensively and with great force. The pain intensifies rapidly and interferes with the use of the arm and it may also radiate down the lateral side and back of the forearm. It is relieved by rest but returns when the arm is again used.

Upon palpation, the pain is accurately localized over the posterior aspect of the radial-humeral articulation and is easily located by comparing it with the normal arm or joint which will show a much deeper dimple or depression than the affected one will. Extension and pronation are slightly restricted and painful. X-ray examination will prove negative.

TREATMENT: A specific adjustment upon the radial-humeral articulation will, in many cases, give dramatic relief and also restore normal movement to the joint (Fig. 102). This correction is made gently but with a quick, short thrust, and it is essential that the patient's muscles be relaxed. In mildly strained or subluxated articulations, such as those presented by stenographers, this move causes very little discomfort. However, when there is a severe misalignment and tissues must be freed, this move can be somewhat painful for two or three seconds. It should not be used in the advanced stages of adhesions where the elbow cannot be straightened, or in cases of osteoarthritis.

Caution should also be remembered where there is a possibility of ulnar subluxation or dislocation to the superior. Such an injury can be caused by a fall in which the arm is extended at the time of impact.

Therefore, when in doubt, the use of x-ray films is necessary in order to confirm or eliminate the presence of a superior subluxation, dislocation or fracture.

THE ULNAR SUBLUXATION

This injury usually occurs following a fall in which the arm was extended in the hope of breaking the force of the impact. In these instances, x-ray films should be taken of both elbows for comparative purposes. The ulnar subluxation is usually to the superior and this can readily be seen on the comparative films.

CORRECTION: The adjustment given for this correction is not usually painful (Fig. 107). This move has a beneficial effect on both the ulna and the radius and gives relief in the articular conditions of the elbow.

The three following situations will be discussed briefly so that the busy doctor will have a quick reference concerning these pathologies which are not likely to respond to adjustments but of which he must be aware in order to give correct advice to the patient. Specific adjustment of the articulation is, in the writer's opinion, not warranted in the following types of pathologies. However, if the doctor wishes to use conservative treatment, such as heat, mild massage or spinal adjustments, some relief may be given to the patient and each doctor will have to evaluate the individual case.

OSTEOARTHRITIS OF THE ELBOW JOINT

This is a relatively uncommon situation because the elbow is not a weight bearing articulation. The symptoms are chiefly located in the radio-humeral joint and are most often caused by injury, generally the aftermath of a fracture. However, oft repeated minor trauma, overuse or misuse, such as that sustained by those who work with air hammers, or anything that causes repeated jarring, can have a gradual adverse effect. The symptoms are intermittent pain and limitation of movement with pain being felt only on the extreme range of joint movement. Locking of the articulation due to the presence of a loose body is sometimes the first symptom to attract attention.

THE SUPERIOR ULNAR SUBLUXATION

When making this correction, the arm should NEVER be fully extended because of possible damage to the tip of the olecranon process. X-ray films should be made to eliminate the possibility of fracture.

When making this adjustment, contact should never be taken directly upon the ulna. Have the patient sit on a stool on one side of the adjusting table and lay his arm across it with the elbow partially flexed. The doctor sits on the opposite side and places his left hand in the joint as shown in Fig. 107, and with his right hand he encircles the wrist just above the joint. Moderate traction is then applied to remove the slack from the muscles and tendons. At this point the thrust is given, the doctor moving his left hand into the

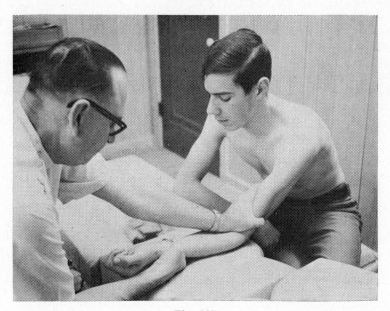

Fig. 107

joint and toward the patient while simultaneously pulling the distal end of the forearm toward himself. Reverse the positioning of the hands for adjusting the right arm.

PERIARTICULAR OSSIFICATION

Periarticular ossification is common after any injury to a joint, particularly the elbow. The injury causes a hematoma, the periosteum is lifted from the bone and ossification occurs beneath the hematoma. After a time, the ossification consolidates and is radiologically demonstrable. The chief symptom is the limitation of movement which at first is considerable. It is not unusual to have flexion and extension nearly absent and gross restriction after a severe injury is a warning that ossification may be taking place which, in turn, can produce much permanent limitation.

OSTEOCHONDRITIS DISSICANS

In this particular difficulty the elbow is affected more frequently than any other articulation except the knee, and, because it is difficult to demonstrate by x-ray, is often overlooked. It is most common in young persons between the ages of 15 and 18.

A small, circular portion of the articular cartilage, together with a flake of underlying bone is separated from the rest of the bone and becomes a loose body in the joint. The usual site is the lower aspect of the humerus and that part of the head of the radius which is in contact with the ulna when the forearm is supinated.

The symptoms are moderate pain, limitation of movement, loss of power and locking when the fragment is completely detached. The onset is gradual and seldom is there a history of injury. The diagnosis is made radiologically and, since the condition is difficult to show, several films must be made at various angles.

LOOSE BODIES

These may be caused by osteochondritis dissicans, osteoarthritis or by a detached fragment of the articular cartilage. Multiple loose bodies may be due to synovial osteochondromatosis. The onset is usually gradual with increasing stiffness, loss of power, pain after use along with locking and unlocking, the last mentioned being more frequent when the loose body is situated at the posterior part of the articulation than when it is in front because, in that location, it can be tucked away in the coronoid fossa and give infrequent difficulty.

Chapter XI

DISORDERS OF THE WRIST AND HAND

The functions of the hands are of such great importance that good case management must be exercised in all injuries of the wrist, hand and fingers. Even though they may appear minor, these injuries could have serious results at a later time.

THE SPRAINED WRIST

The sprained or strained wrist is perhaps the most common condition that a chiropractic doctor will come in contact with when treating injuries of this area. A strained or sprained wrist is quite common in athletics and also appears very frequently in occupational pursuits. The history is usually that of a fall on the hand with the arm outstretched, causing pain, disability and swelling. If the doctor is at the scene of the accident or sees the patient shortly thereafter, cold should be applied by way of immersing the hand and wrist in ice water or the use of an ice pack. Ethyl chloride is also very effective.

All sprained wrists should be x-rayed and films should be taken in various planes since a fracture of the scaphoid can easily be overlooked. These fractures seldom unite if left untreated and if left in that state, the symptoms do subside but the area will become a site for possible future arthritis. If a fracture is found, it is best to refer the patient to a specialist in this type of work. If the films are fracture negative, support the wrist with a strong application of tape as shown in Figs. 112 to 116 inclusive.

The usual severely sprained wrist will always be accompanied by subluxations of one or more of the carpal bones along with a subluxation of the radius in its alignment with the carpal bones and the ulna. There may or may not be swelling when the patient comes to the office, depending upon the elapsed time between the injury and time of treatment. However, there will be complaint of pain on certain movements of the hand and wrist required in many of the most common duties pertaining to his occupation.

Even if some time has elapsed since the accident occurred, x-rays should be taken to eliminate a possible hidden fracture or the beginnings of arthritis. It is of paramount importance to locate all subluxations. The writer has had many cases of this type where the accident had taken place two or three months before treatment was instituted. These patients had previously sought help but had been told that nothing was wrong other than a common sprain and that it would simply take time to heal. In a number of these instances the wrist had a spreading appearance and looked much wider than the normal wrist. This, of course, was due to the bony subluxation and lack of integrity of the ligaments surrounding the area. Upon palpation, the subluxated bones can easily be located. Pain will be elicited upon pressure over the affected carpal bones and adjacent tissues. In practically all cases the radius is subluxated along with the carpal bones.

All subluxations must be adjusted. The method shown in Figs. 109, 110 and 111 is for the carpals while the radial correction is shown in Fig. 102 in the discussion of the elbow. After the adjustment a strong taping must be applied as shown in Figs. 112-116. If the skin becomes irritated from the tape, a fabric splint device must be substituted. This is available at any drug store. Usually three to five adjustments over a period of from two to three weeks is required, at which time the patient should be pain free.

THE STRAINED WRIST

This is usually caused by overuse or misuse and should be taped in the same manner as the sprained wrist except that the tape is placed four to six inches higher up the arm, depending upon the size of the tender area, than the taped area in a sprain. Subluxations of the carpal bones are quite frequent and these should be located and adjusted if present. Again, the doctor should not neglect to check the patient for a possible radial subluxation. Since this condition overlaps with occupational tenosynovitis, it will be discussed further under that heading in the following paragraphs.

OCCUPATIONAL TENOSYNOVITIS

Acute tenosynovitis of occupational origin is, at first glance, a seemingly trivial condition. It has become common in these days of assembly line production where an employee must repeatedly perform the same movements at a hurried pace in order to keep up with the line. The strain on certain muscles in this repetitive action may cause irritation to the involved tendons and their sheaths, and is responsible for the loss of a considerable number of working hours. This common complaint nearly always involves the extensors and the two areas that can be defined are:

1. The musculotendinous junction in the lower region of the back of the forearm. The muscles affected are the extensors of the wrist, mainly on the radial side of the arm, and the abductors of the thumb.

2. The extensors of the fingers on the back of the hand, most often the extensors of the forefingers. However, any of the other tendons may be involved alone or simultaneously.

There are four known causes for this disorder.

1. Repeated rapid movements along with pressure such as the squeezing of a tool handle. Very often this will occur when returning to work after an absence from it during which time the muscles have become unaccustomed to the strain. It may also result from an increase in work speed or work hours.

2. An injury such as receiving a blow on the tendon. This produces immediate pain which worsens during the ensuing days. In such an instance, cold should be applied at once and heat may be used after 24 hours. In all cases, the tendons should be immobilized by a strong taping or efficient wrapping.

3. Strain due to the overstretching of tendons, most often at the site of the musculotendinous junction.

4. Benign tumors, or at times, a ganglion presses on a tendon and interferes with free movement. Only rarely will interference be caused by a small fibroma or synovioma.

SYMPTOMS. Pain will be noted in the region of the affected tendon or muscle in the hand or lower part of the forearm and will radiate over a wide area. There may be some swelling which is more visible when the lesion is in the forearm. Very often there is crepitus which can be felt and also heard on osculation along with tenderness on pressure over the affected area.

Years ago, before farming became so completely mechanized, the writer would see a great number of these cases, particularly in the fall when corn was being hand husked. The patient, if he had not sought help previously, would always come in with his own diagnosis of a sprained wrist, and if he had received professional advice, the mis-diagnoses were surprisingly frequent. Only rarely was it correctly labeled as an occupational tenosynovitis.

TREATMENT. With proper case management, recovery is fairly rapid. First, a strong taping must be applied as shown in Figs. 112

to 116 and the hand must have rest for a week to ten days. In the majority of cases, the carpals and the radius will present misalignments and these should be adjusted as soon as the patient's tolerance will permit, unless an arthritic situation intervenes. After four or five days, the tape should be removed and the muscles and tendons gently stretched by bending the hand back and forth after which the tape is reapplied. If the skin should be too irritated to tolerate more tape, a wrist support must be applied which should be worn until recovery is complete.

THE ADJUSTMENT OF THE SPRAINED OR STRAINED WRIST

In nearly all sprained wrists there will be a subluxation of one or more of the carpal bones. These must be adjusted and the ligaments supported with tape.

In Fig. 109 the wrist is palpated for tenderness and specific subluxations and the doctor's crossed thumbs placed over the misaligned bone. The wrist is then manipulated from side to side holding firm pressure over the subluxation (Figs. 110 and 111). Then a downward pressure is used which will raise the palm of the hand slightly higher than shown in Fig. 109. In all cases of sprained wrists, the radius should be checked for subluxation and corrected if found.

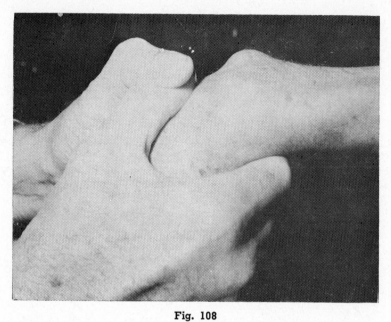

Fig. 108

WRONG WAY. Never, never manipulate a wrist with the hand pointing downward. Wrong way.

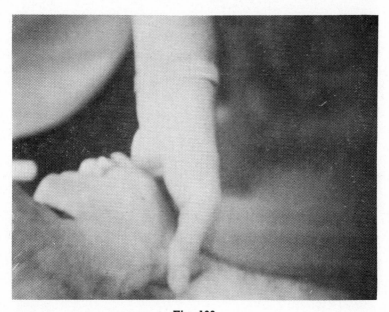

Fig. 109

CORRECT WAY. Note that the patient's palm is slightly above the level of the forearm with the fingers relaxed.

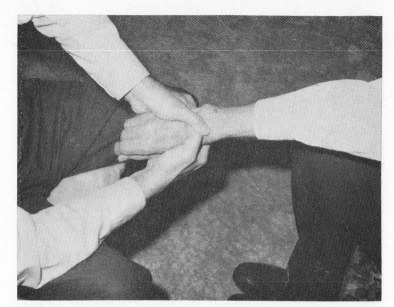

Fig. 110

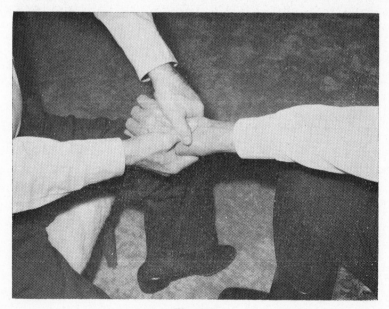

Fig. 111

234

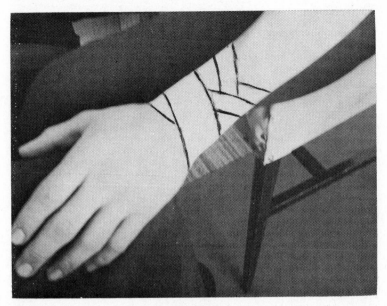

Fig. 112

TAPING OF THE WRIST

In the above photograph the first application of tape is shown. The hand is placed on the doctor's knee so that the hand and fingers are elevated and the wrist drops lower. This will allow the tendons to relax, compress the carpal bones, and, after the taping, will cause pressure on the area when the wrist is bent. Four pieces are criss-crossed over the wrist as shown. Do not enclose the underside of the wrist with this tape.

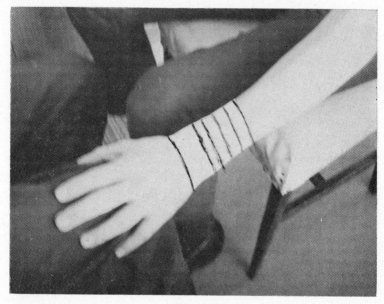

Fig. 113

This picture shows five or six strips of tape placed horizontally over the criss-crossed pieces. These strips are applied snugly, with the hand still in the original position, and they must be short enough not to encircle the wrist.

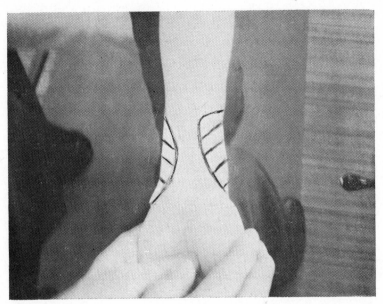

Fig. 114

This picture shows the opening on the underside of the wrist.

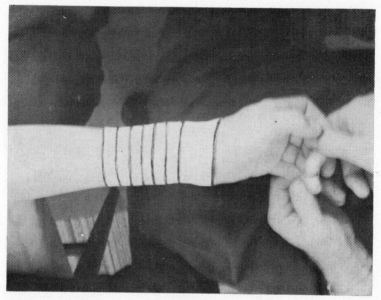

Fig. 115

This photograph shows the underside of the wrist with seven or eight pieces of tape applied over the opening. The reason for using the short pieces of tape is not to inhibit circulation. If strips were used that were long enough to encircle the articulation, these would almost invariably cause severe swelling.

238

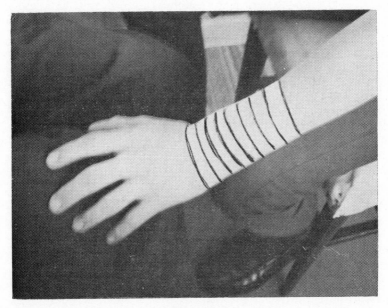

Fig. 116

The final step is shown in the above photograph and consists of applying another layer in the same manner as in Fig. 113 except that several more tape strips are used, seven or eight. The writer has found that inch and a half wide tape is the most versatile in these tapings.

SPRAINS OF THE METACARPO-PHALANGEAL JOINTS

These injuries occur as the result of a severe lateral force or from sudden hyperextension. There is considerable pain and disability. Recovery is slow and the patient finds it difficult to understand why the finger or thumb is not normal since he almost always considers the injury very minor and will usually wait a month or six weeks before seeking help.

In all of these injuries there is a subluxation which must be corrected (Figs. 125, 126, 127 and 133). Thereafter, supportive measures must be applied, either taping or splinting as shown in Figs. 123 and 130, depending upon the severity of the injury. The adjustment and supportive measures may have to be repeated several times, until the ligaments have regained their integrity.

Rupture of the lateral ligament of the thumb is the most troublesome of these injuries. The thumb will be found to be weak and unstable with unnatural mobility. In case of a complete rupture, the patient should be sent to an orthopedic surgeon for repairs.

SPRAINS OF THE INTERPHALANGEAL JOINTS

The delicate capsule and collateral ligaments of these small, slender articulations are easily sprained or torn and they are frequently dislocated. The ligaments may be torn or a bone fragment avulsed.

These injuries are more serious than is generally admitted even when the ligaments are only sprained. Very often they are left untreated and the finger remains crippled for months. Most patients, and even many professionals, dismiss it as trivial and say that it will take care of itself. Again, the writer wishes to point out that in a sprain there is nearly always a subluxation which must be corrected. Supportive measures must be used to restore ligamentous integrity. The methods shown in Figs. 120 to 123 are to be used EXCEPT without the upward pull, OR in milder sprains, the method shown in Fig. 132.

SITUATIONS TO BE RECOGNIZED

The following four conditions are generally not chiropractic cases but they should nevertheless be recognized so that proper treatment can be suggested. For that reason they are being described.

CHRONIC INFLAMMATORY TENOSYNOVITIS
The palmar bursa, which is the sheath surrounding the flexor tendon at the wrist, when distended, causes the transverse carpal

ligament to form a constriction across the center area so that a swelling will appear both above and below the ligament and into the palm. The term "compound palmar ganglion" is often used to describe any swelling of this nature. The synovial sheath is greatly thickened and convoluted and usually there is a thick, fibrinous deposit adherent to both layers of the sheath, encircling each tendon separately. Sometimes there are typical "melon seed" bodies.

The signs and symptoms resemble those of tuberculous tenosynovitis so closely that they cannot be differentiated clinically and it can be diagnosed with certainty only after a complete histological and bacteriological examination. The method of treatment is to remove the affected synovial sheath by dissection. This gives generally good results unless a rheumatoid condition is present to complicate matters.

TUBERCULAR TENOSYNOVITIS

Tubercular tenosynovitis is a disease of adult life which affects the tendons and sheaths of the hands, more often the flexors than the extensors. Infection of the right hand is more common than the left and it occurs very frequently in craftsmen who work with their hands.

The infection commences in the synovial sheath, most generally in the palm of the hand, and is of low virulence. It spreads slowly until the radial and ulnar bursae and their extensors are involved, then proceeds into the area of the forearm until the fingers may finally become involved. The onset is insidious and the history may extend over a year or two. The first complaint is of a gradual swelling and stiffness of the fingers. Later the loss of power becomes marked and the fingers are held in a semiflexed position and they can be neither fully flexed or fully extended. Pain in the forearm or palm is seldom present but there may be numbness and tingling in the thumb and fingers due to compression of the median nerve. The diagnosis must be soundly based before a biopsy is recommended and surgery advised.

STENOSING TENOVAGINITIS (HOFFMAN'S DISEASE)

This is a fairly frequent condition in which there is a thickening of the common sheath of the abductor pollicis longus and the extensor pollicis brevis tendons which lie on the lateral side of the lower end of the radius. It is seen more frequently in women than in men and the etiology is unknown but it is thought that repeated minor stress and strain is a contributing factor. The complaint is

most often seen in persons whose occupation involves strong gripping by a partially abducted thumb, such as one would use in a
wringing or twisting motion.

Symptoms. Pain is felt at the lateral side of the wrist, radiating
up the forearm and down the thumb. It is aggravated by the use
of the hand and gradually worsens until there is considerable disability. Generally the onset of symptoms is gradual though occasionally it is abrupt and follows a minor strain or injury.

Treatment. Surprisingly, neither rest, supportive measures or
physiotherapy seems to be the answer. The pain may be relieved
temporarily but returns quickly when the part is used despite the
fact that the symptoms appeared slowly. When the onset of pain
is abrupt and follows strain or injury, the wrist and thumb should
be supported and subluxations of the carpal bones, radius and
thumb should be corrected if present. The thumb is adjusted by
expansion of the articulation as shown in Fig. 127. In the absence of
any kind of strain or injury, a simple surgical procedure gives the
quickest relief by excision of the thickened segment.

TRIGGER FINGER (SNAPPING FINGER)

This is a difficulty in which the fibrous sheath covering the
flexor tendons of one of the fingers or thumb becomes thickened
in a manner closely resembling stenosing tenovaginitis. The lesion,
which is usually at the level of the metacarpal-phalangeal joint,
presents the following conditions:

1. A thickening and stenosis of the tendon sheath and

2. A small nodule which forms in the tendon sheath distal to
   the thickening causes the tendon to become bunched up by
   the squeezing action of the constricted sheath.

The lesion may occur at any age but is most usually found during infancy or middle age, the thumb being most generally affected
in babies and the ring or middle fingers in adults. Usually only one
finger is affected but in rare instances, several fingers of one or
both hands are involved.

The patient often does not realize what is happening and will
point out some other part of the finger as the offending area. The
nodule on the tendon can be palpated when the examining finger
is placed over it and the patient instructed to flex and extend the
finger. The condition can be corrected by a fairly simple surgical
procedure.

THE GANGLION

A ganglion is a cystic swelling occurring in association with a joint or tendon sheath. It has a fibrous outer coat and an inner synovial layer closely resembling the articular synovial membrane and contains a thick, gelatinous fluid. Some pathologists regard ganglia as herniations of the tendon sheaths or joints. There is a close relationship between ganglia and bursae and it is often difficult to draw a distinct division between them. Ganglia occur most frequently around the wrists and hands, at times in the ankle and foot. They are at least five times more common on the dorsal surface than on the ventral. Usually they grow slowly but on occasion may appear very suddenly. The chief symptom is a localized swelling. There may be weakness in the grip of the hand accompanied by aching and at times there is pain from pressure on adjacent tendons or nerves. A common site for a small ganglion is deep under the extensor tendons on the back of the wrist which will interfere considerably with the functions of the hand.

The majority of patients with this difficulty are women. The writer has had quite a number of cases which occurred in salesladies. All had a similar case history, namely, while trying to make a sale of a winter coat, they were required to take down and replace twenty or more heavy garments from the racks. This caused the ganglion to appear, apparently from the strain of the twisting action on the hand and wrist along with the weight of the garments. Another common cause is found in homemakers who do a great deal of canning or hand laundry.

TREATMENT. The simplest treatment is to try to break the ganglion by a firm contact and pressure. The same contact is applied as that which is used to adjust the subluxated wrist bones (Fig. 109). To prevent the recurrence of the ganglion, place a piece of chiropodists felt over it. Next, place a penny on the felt directly over the ganglion so that a constant pressure can be exerted by the application of tape (Fig. 117). The taping procedure is the same as that used in a sprained wrist (Figs. 112 to 116).

If the adjustment and pressure procedure is not successful in dispersing the fluid, place the felt, penny and pressure taping anyway since many of these conditions will disappear with the use of supportive and pressure measures alone. If no chiropodists felt is available, fold several thicknesses of gauze and place the penny on it, criss-crossing the penny with two bandaids and then applying the pressure taping over the whole wrist.

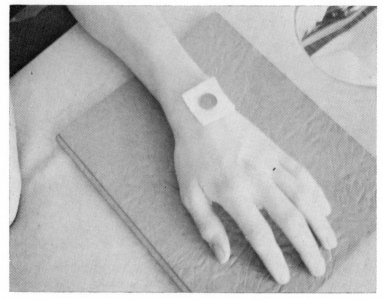

Fig. 117

CARE OF THE GANGLION

The wrist is adjusted as shown in Fig. 109 with firm pressure on the ganglion. Then a piece of chiropodist's felt is placed on it and a penny put on the felt directly over the ganglion. Then the regular taping for a sprained wrist is applied with firm pressure, as outlined in Figs. 112 to 116.

THE MALLET FINGER

Tendons of the hand are susceptible to severe sprains and tears and the four tendons of the extensor digitorum communis are particularly vulnerable. These sprains and tears are usually caused by the finger being struck on its end with a ball in games such as basketball, baseball, football and volleyball. However, it may also occur spontaneously or from trivial violence and the patient is unable to name a particular cause except to say that "it happened at work." The writer has had two cases where the patient was merely putting her coat on and in the act of running her hand through the sleeve, the tendon was injured and a mallet finger resulted. Whether the gentlemen helping the ladies with their coats became overenthusiastic is a possibility since both of them were young and unmarried!

The mallet finger deformity may be caused by—

1. A tear of the tendon immediately proximal to its insertion and is caused by an incoordinated contraction of the muscles. As mentioned, it may follow a trivial injury or appear to be of spontaneous origin.

2. Avulsion of the extensor tendon from its insertion into the base of the terminal phalanx, either with or without an attached fragment of bone. It is usually due to a severe blow on the fingertip, flexing it forcibly at the moment when the extensor tendon is contracted, such as in the act of catching a ball.

After the injury, the finger assumes a position of about 70% of flexion at the terminal interphalangeal joint (Fig. 118). It cannot actively be extended but can be moved to normal position with help. However, when the assistance is released, it returns to its abnormal position. Even though it may not particularly interfere with work, it is nonetheless an inconvenience and an annoyance because the finger will catch on certain objects.

TREATMENT. There is no need to try adjustive procedures in this situation. The best way to attempt correction is through supportive measures. The writer has cared for a goodly number of these cases since it is a frequent injury in athletics. By following the outlined procedures, good results may be obtained.

For splints, the writer has found that ordinary paper clips make an excellent device. To make them comfortable, they must be covered with tape as shown in Fig. 119, using one-half or three-quarter inch tape both for the clips as well as for taping the finger.

1. Prepare the clips and cut the patient's fingernail very short.

2. Place a piece of tape on the finger that is cut long enough to extend from just below the middle joint of the injured finger on the palmar side, over the end of it and back down to just below the middle articulation on the opposite side of the finger (Fig. 120).

3. Place the prepared splints as shown in Fig. 121.

4. Next, place another piece of tape as described in step 2, Fig. 122.

5. Then tear short strips of tape to encircle the finger as shown in Fig. 123. NOTE: The encircling tape strips must be applied with very LIGHT pressure so that circulation is not inhibited. The writer has always been very emphatic about avoiding encirclement of an articulation if it is at all possible. This is an exception and therefore the cautionary statement of using light pressure on the encircling strips, though the splints do aid in the prevention of circulatory stasis.

The splints should remain in place for about a week and then checked. If it is fairly well improved, retape as described in step 2 above, and use only one encircling strip at the middle articulation. If improvement is only slight, retape completely using the splints again. Usually within about three weeks the finger will be nearly normal though there still may be some extensor lag. This will improve in a few more weeks. In a few cases the deformity will not disappear completely but will give no difficulty in the pursuit of normal duties. Operative repair of the tendon seldom gives any results and in long standing injuries, very little can be done.

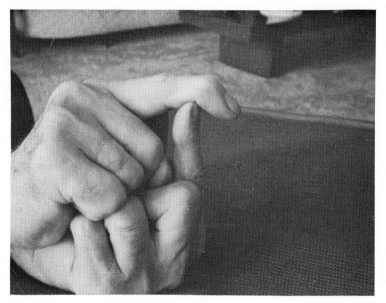

Fig. 118
This picture simulates the appearance of a mallet finger.

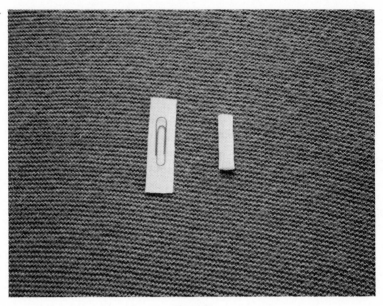

Fig. 119

Here are shown the paper clips which are covered with tape and used as splints. The tape is torn lengthwise as described in Fig. 120.

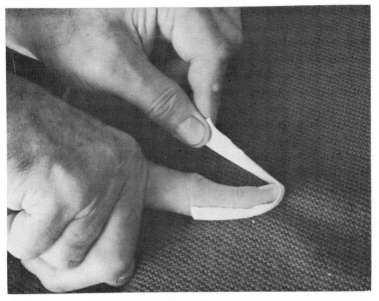

Fig. 120

Tear a strip of tape long enough to reach around the end of the finger from middle joint to middle joint, with enough pressure over the end of the finger to straighten it. Use inch and a half tape which is torn in half **lengthwise** for finger tapings, or especially cut one-half inch tape.

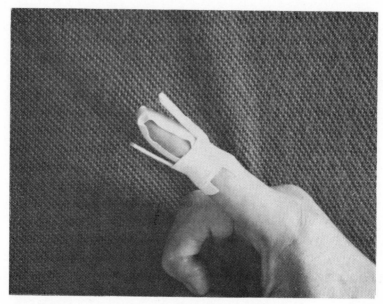

Fig. 121

Here the splints are shown in place, held by an encircling tape strip. Note: Put only enough tension on this encircling strip to hold the splints. It is the only time the writer uses an encircling piece of tape.

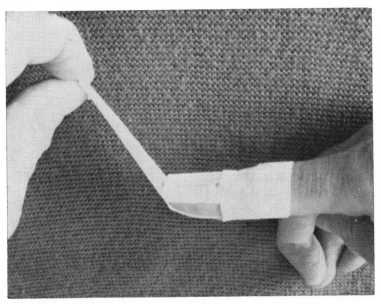

Fig. 122

With the splints lying closely against the finger, cover them with another strip of tape in the same manner as in Fig. 120.

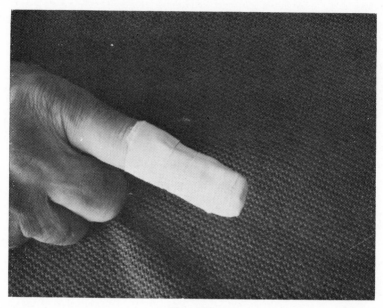

Fig. 123

This is the completed taping using encircling strips that have been applied with light pressure. Note: VERY light pressure so that circulation is not inhibited.

RUPTURE OF THE POLLICIS LONGUS

Rupture of the tendon of this muscle takes place where it lies in a groove on the back of the lower portion of the radius and usually appears in a manner that is considered spontaneous. It often follows an injury to the lower end of the radius and occurs, in most cases, after a latent period of several months. It may also occur in persons with a history of long standing rheumatoid arthritis when the rupture will appear to follow a sprained wrist. X-rays usually show evidence of an old fracture. The tendon becomes frayed at the site of fracture and then may rupture from a trifling incident. When the basic and underlying cause is rheumatoid arthritis, the patient may be unaware of what happened to produce his awkwardness in the use of the thumb until he consults a doctor.

The sign of the lesion is an inability to extend the thumb normally at the interphalangeal joint. Surgery is advised in younger persons, but when the hands are arthritic, it should not be attempted since no appreciable results will be evident.

THE BUTTON-HOLE DEFORMITY

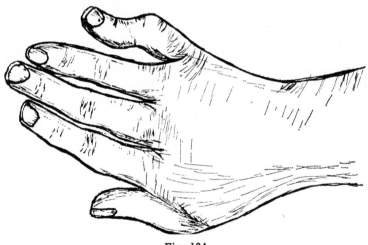

Fig. 124

This situation is caused by a tear of the central slip of the tendon at the level of the proximal interphalangeal joint. It may occur as the result of violence but most often from a cut with a knife. Surgery is generally recommended for this condition, however, results are uncertain.

DISLOCATIONS OF THE THUMB AND INTERPHALANGEAL JOINTS

Dislocations of these articulations are quite common, especially in athletics where the thumb seems to receive more than its share. Persons who are in occupations where they must handle heavy tools are often vulnerable to these injuries, however, any sudden blow can cause them.

Not long ago the writer had an unusual and interesting case in this category—unusual because of the severity of the dislocation and interesting because of the way in which he received the injury. He was a high school junior and was teasing a girl in the school hallway between classes when the girl took one of her books and tried to give him a "bop" on the head. He raised his hand to ward off the blow and the book struck his middle finger, driving the middle phalanx down over the proximal one nearly to the joint. Since he was a star basketball player, his coach brought him in at once. The finger appeared an inch shorter than the middle and ring fingers and he was in great pain. His finger was adjusted as shown in Fig. 131, and a splint was applied. The splint was made by cutting a tongue depressor in half after preparing it as shown in Fig. 37, padding it well with cotton and applying it to the finger with tape, as shown in Figs. 121, 122 and 123. He was asked to return in a week, at which time the splint was removed and the middle and ring fingers were taped together as shown in Fig. 132, the ring finger acting as a mild splint. After two more weeks, the finger appeared to be completely healed and he had no further difficulty.

The doctor must bear in mind that these injuries are very painful and therefore, when making the adjustment, great care must be taken to have the proper contact, to have it firm yet gentle and to get it done on the first attempt. The docor must have complete control of the entire hand area or he may slip on the contact. In giving this adjustment, traction is not held as in a shoulder dislocation. Rather, it is done by a quick, strong pull. Because the patient is in much pain, it is best, if possible, to have him lying down while making the correction.

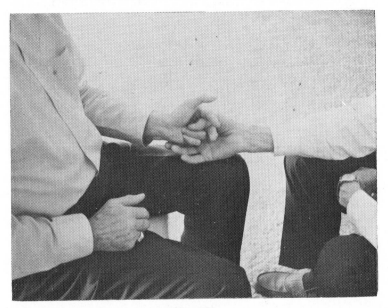

Fig. 125

This picture shows the beginning of the contact in the reduction of a dislocation or sprain. The patient should be either sitting on a stool or lying on the adjusting table. The doctor's index and middle fingers are placed across the patient's injured thumb at a point midway between the two joints.

255

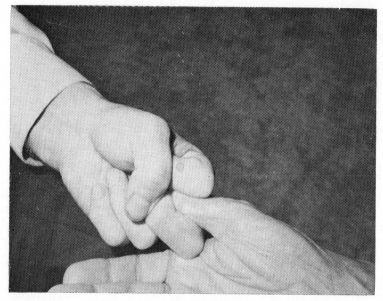

Fig. 126

The doctor then bends his two fingers sharply around the patient's thumb and crosses his bent fingers with his bent thumb as shown. This produces a very firm contact on the injured member and avoids slippage which would be very painful to the patient.

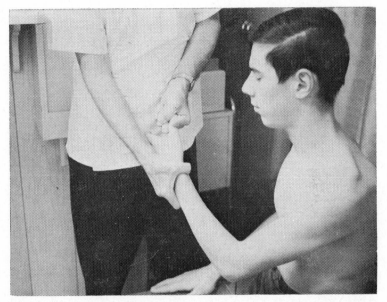

Fig. 127

The above photograph shows how the doctor steadies the patient's hand with his other hand grasping around the wrist joint proper. Do NOT hold it above the articulation. With the patient's hand thus steadied, the doctor gives a fast, firm, short and straight pull toward himself. In making this correction, the doctor may either stand or sit since the leverage in either position is the same.

In the case of sprains, the subluxation will be either lateral-superior, superior or medial superior and the doctor uses the same contact as is used for the dislocation. However, he varies the line of pull slightly according to the subluxation present, namely, straight toward himself for the superior one, toward and slightly lateral for the lateral one and toward and slightly medial for the medial misalignment.

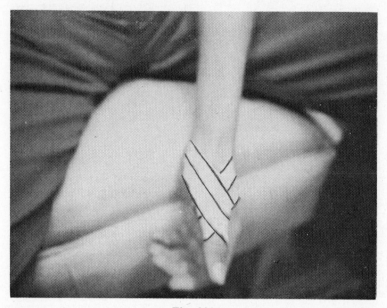

Fig. 128

The above photograph shows the first step in the taping. Two or three strips of one inch wide tape are applied in the criss-cross manner, each strip being four or five inches long. The tape is applied starting at the under or palmar side of the thumb, then running diagonally so they will cross over the injured articulation. The strips do join on the palmar side of the thumb.

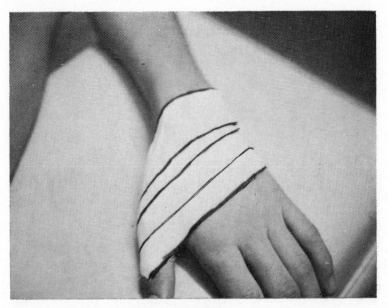

Fig. 129

This is the second step where the strips are run diagonally from the lateral margin of the hand to just a little beyond the medial margin of the thumb and wrist. Four or five strips are used.

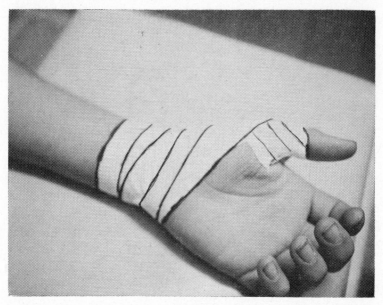

Fig. 130

Here is shown the completed taping after the third tape application has been made. These strips run somewhat diagonally from the medial side of the thumb to the lateral side of the hand, covering the ends of the tape applied in step two.

ADJUSTING THE SPRAINED OR DISLOCATED MEDIAL PHALANGEAL ARTICULATIONS

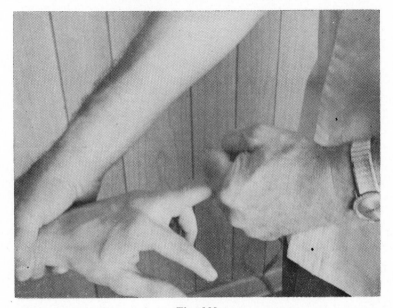

Fig. 131

When adjusting the middle articulation of any of the fingers, the same contacts are used as shown in Figs. 125 and 126, on the thumb, except, of course, that the contact point is between the distal and medial articulations of the fingers. The adjustive directional pull is the same as described under the thumb.

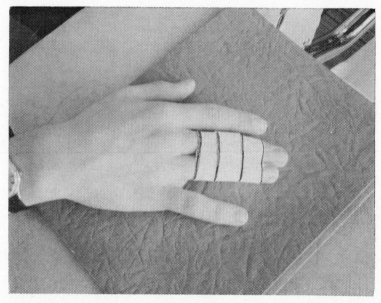

Fig. 132

This photograph shows a method of using a neighboring finger as a splint to protect the injured one. It is used in joint injuries such as sprains and strains that are not severe enough to require complete splinting, or also in the latter stages of supporting a dislocated joint when the full splint is no longer necessary.

To apply a complete splint, prepare a tongue depressor as shown in Fig. 37 and cut it in half. Then cover the cut edge with a bit of tape to prevent the rough edge from injuring the skin. One-half of this splint is applied to the palmar side of the finger with the foam side against the skin and is taped in place with encircling strips, being SURE that they are not tight enough to inhibit circulation. In severe injuries, the other half of the splint is applied to the top of the finger, then both are taped to the finger at the same time.

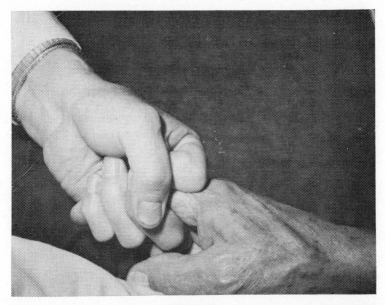

Fig. 133

The above picture shows the contact when adjusting the metacarpophalangeal articulation. The contact, adjustment and directional adjustive pull is the same as that used for the thumb shown in Figs. 126 and 127, except that instead of making the contact midway between the two articulations, this one is made as close as possible to the injured joint.

Support should be applied by way of taping the injured finger to its neighbor and running two strips of tape, one on top of the other, around the hand and directly over the knuckles, using inch and a half tape. Or, if the doctor wishes, he may apply a shaped metal or hard plastic wrist-hand splint available at a drug store.

Chapter XII

SHOULDER AND ARM EXERCISES

Exercises are very important for the purpose of restoring muscular and ligamentous tone after injury, in the treatment of bursitis, the frozen shoulder, tenosynovitis, etc.

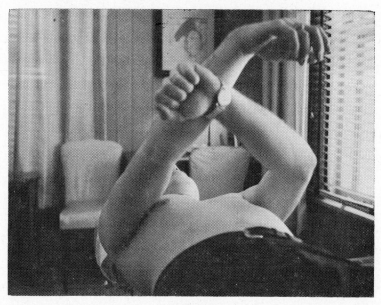

Fig. 134

The above photograph and the following one are exercises that are to be suggested as the initial ones in really severe situations and also after a subglenoid dislocation. These are to be done while lying on the back in bed. When the patient is unable to raise the injured arm, have him raise it to his tolerance with the uninjured one as shown. The injured arm should be raised and lowered a number of times—to his tolerance—in each exercise "period," at least several a day. He can also gradually rotate the arm inward from this position.

264

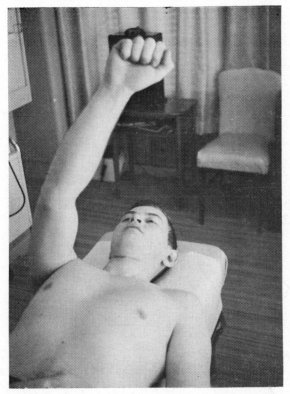

Fig. 135

If the patient can raise his arm to some extent, start him as shown above, raising the arm, then gradually rotating it inward and outward. This again should be repeated several times daily to his tolerance.

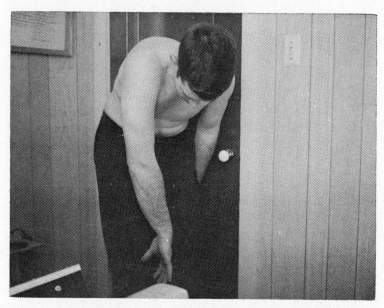

Fig. 136

Above is pictured a mild exercise particularly suitable for use after dislocations, frozen shoulder and bursitis. The patient is instructed to bend forward slightly and rotate the arm, first in small circles, later in larger ones with particular emphasis on the inward rotation.

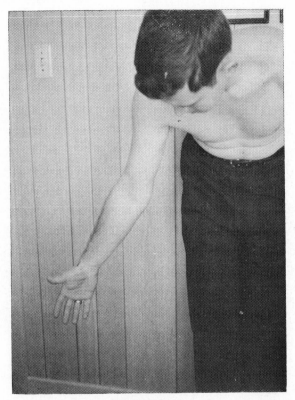

Fig. 137

The photograph shows a similar position except that the arm is rotated outwardly. Do NOT suggest this exercise after an anterior dislocation and NEITHER the above one or the previously shown one after a subglenoid dislocation.

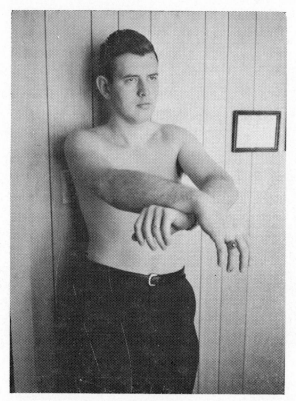

Fig. 138

This photograph and the following one show the mild exercise with support in the upright position. In this posture it takes a great deal more muscular effort than when the patient is lying on his back and has the stabilizing effect of body weight on the back muscles. Therefore, the severely injured person will progress to this stage after starting as in Fig. 134 and those who can tolerate to start in the standing posture may do so. They are to be instructed to raise the injured arm as high as tolerable and then easily move it from side to side.

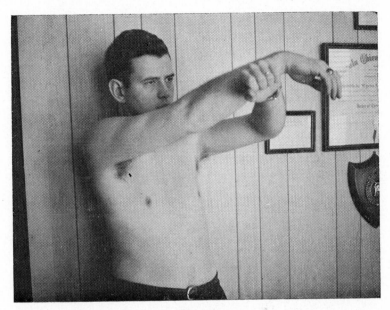

Fig. 139

The higher that the patient can raise his arm for this exercise, the more beneficial it will be.

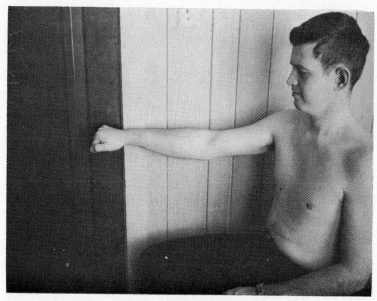

Fig. 140

Another beneficial exercise is to have the patient sit so that when his arm is raised as shown, it is parallel with a doorknob. He should grasp it and lean back with his body weight, up to his tolerance of stretch.

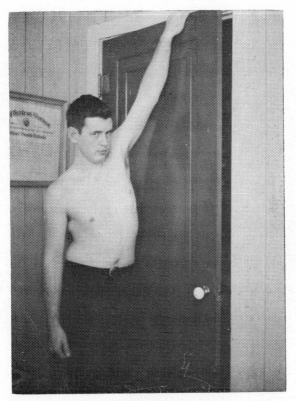

Fig. 141

In the later stages of healing, the patient should be instructed to raise the arm high as shown and to let part of his body weight down, again stretching the area to his tolerance. This particular exercise is excellent in cases of tenosynovitis after the patient has progressed far enough not to need supportive taping.

The exercises shown here are excellent muscle strengtheners and the patient should be instructed to do them as soon as feasible.

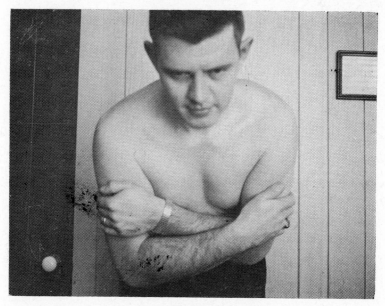

Fig. 142

To further strengthen his muscles, have the patient grasp his arms as shown and exert all possible inward pressure with his muscles.

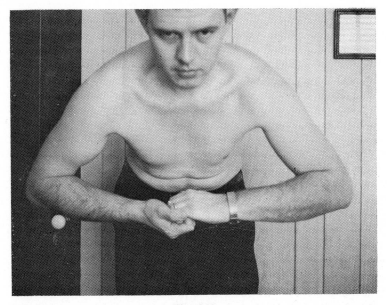

Fig. 143

With the arms and fingers in the position shown, have him exert outward pressure as though trying to pull his hands apart. The last two exercises shown are particularly beneficial for strengthening muscles after all shoulder dislocations, most shoulder syndromes and especially in the frozen shoulder.

CONCLUSION

It is the writer's hope that he has given the practitioner who reads this book some ideas that will be useful to him in caring for the difficult cases that present themselves for treatment involving the shoulder, arm and hand syndrome. It has been his observation in many years of practice and lecturing in many states, that one of the weaknesses in our profession lies in the lack of knowledge and proper case management in the care of dislocations, sprains and strains of the extra-spinal articulations.

In some ways our profession reminds one of the story of Queen Elizabeth of England and Sir Francis Drake. It seems that in Sir Francis Drake's travels, which helped to make England a great power, he came in contact with silk for the first time and brought back a pair of silk stockings for his Queen. These he gave to the lady in waiting to be presented to Her Majesty. The following day he received a curt note which read, "Sir, the Queen of England has no legs." Likewise, too many of our profession practice without giving the extra-spinal articulation their just due when it comes to relieving the many aches, pains and miseries that they can cause.

Important as the spine is, there are other areas in the body where misalignments and muscle contracture can also produce nerve pressure. Most important are the muscles where the neuro-vascular bundles run in close proximity to them and where their bony attachments act either as a roof or floor. Contracture of such muscles can cause compression of important nerve and blood vessel structures and produce as much difficulty as a subluxated vertebra. Where this occurs most frequently is between the first rib and clavicle, between the scalene muscles, the coracoid process and pectoralis minor and the important quadrangular space.

The writer does not claim to have discovered anything new since manipulation for the relief of nerve pressure was practiced many hundreds of years ago. It is, however, his hope to make the profession think and expand work along this line. It cannot be beaten as an efficient and lasting practice builder.

INDEX